CLARK CO

D0405181

About the Authors

MAR - - 2010

VALENTÍN FUSTER, MD, PhD, is director of the Mount Sinai Heart Center in New York City, general director of the National Center for Cardiovascular Investigations (CNIC) in Spain, and former president of the American Heart Association and of the World Heart Federation. His research on causes of coronary disease, which has led to significant advances in the treatment and prevention of heart attacks, has earned him the Príncipe of Asturias Award in 1996. He is the only researcher who has received the highest recognition awards from all five of the most important cardiological institutions: the American Heart Association, the World Heart Federation, the American College of Cardiology, the European Society of Cardiology, and the Inter-American Society of Cardiology. He holds an honorary degree of twenty-six universities around the world.

He is the author of two of the most prestigious books dedicated to clinical cardiology and research, and has offered advice to the *Sesame Street* writers on preventive care to show children how to look after themselves.

JOSEP CORBELLA is a science and health writer based in Barcelona, Spain. He is a staff writer for the daily newspaper *La Vanguardia* and the coauthor of the Spanish bestseller *Sapiens* about human evolution. He has received many awards from medical societies and patient advocacy groups in the fields of cancer, nutrition, and child psychiatry.

LAS VEGAS-CLARK COUNTY
LIBRARY DISTRICT
833 LAS VEGAS BLVD. N
LAS VEGAS, NEVADA 89101

CLARK CO. LIBRARY

THE HEART
MANUAL

THE HEART MANUAL

MY SCIENTIFIC ADVICE FOR EATING BETTER, FEELING BETTER, AND LIVING A STRESS-FREE LIFE NOW

Valentín Fuster, MD, PhD

With the Collaboration of Josep Corbella

Translated from Spanish by
Ted Krasny and Graham Thompson

Foreword by Mehmet C. Oz, MD

Illustrations by Brosmind Studio and Jaime Vicente

HARPER

NEW YORK · LONDON · TORONTO · SYDNEY

HARPER

This book is designed to give information on prevention of medical conditions with emphasis on cardiovascular diseases and on overall health promotion for your personal knowledge and to help you be a more informed consumer of medical and health services. It is not intended to be complete or exhaustive; nor is it a substitute for the advice of your physician. You should consult your physician before beginning any diet, exercise, or health-related program, and for any specific medical condition or problem you may have.

All efforts have been made to ensure the accuracy of the information contained in this book as of the date published. The authors and the publisher expressly disclaim responsibility for any adverse effects arising from the use or application of the information contained herein.

Illustrations on pages 21, 24, 27, 28, 29, 67, 80, 107, 227, 233, and 266 are copyright © 2010 by Brosmind Studio. These illustrations have been reproduced with the permission of Editorial Planeta.
Illustrations on pages 223 and 247 are copyright © 2010 by Jaime Vicente.

Originally published as *La ciencia de la salud* by Editorial Planeta, S.A., in Spain in 2006.

THE HEART MANUAL. Copyright © 2006, 2010 by Valentín Fuster and Josep Corbella. Translation copyright © 2010 by Ted Krasny and Graham Thompson. Foreword copyright © 2010 by Mehmet C. Oz. All rights reserved. Printed in the United States of America. No part of this book may be used or reproduced in any manner whatsoever without written permission except in the case of brief quotations embodied in critical articles and reviews. For information address HarperCollins Publishers, 10 East 53rd Street, New York, NY 10022.

HarperCollins books may be purchased for educational, business, or sales promotional use. For information please write: Special Markets Department, HarperCollins Publishers, 10 East 53rd Street, New York, NY 10022.

FIRST EDITION

Designed by Justin Dodd

Library of Congress Cataloging-in-Publication Data has been applied for.

ISBN 978-0-06-176591-9

10 11 12 13 14   OV/RRD   10 9 8 7 6 5 4 3 2 1

Contents

Foreword

Like many American physicians, I first learned of Valentín Fuster by listening to his captivating lectures. His teachings were reinforced by the generation of cutting edge, caring physicians honored to report that they were trained by Fuster. And, in case a health-care provider might have missed his tsunami of publications, one cannot travel through the hallowed halls of academic medicine and not be influenced by his many peer-reviewed manuscripts and textbooks.

Fuster is a dedicated, caring physician to kings and paupers. He is the chair of one of the most prestigious medical facilities in the nation. He has played leading roles in shaping national policy on more than one continent, and yet he is approachable to all his students.

Fuster has done it all—almost. With this wonderful book, Fuster finally closes the loop with the lay public. In this comprehensive yet accessible tome, Fuster teaches all of us the secrets that he has painstakingly shared with his patients for more than half a century. After a remarkable success in Spanish, Fuster's first language, we are now blessed with an English edition that will help all of us understand the subtle insights needed to become the world expert on ones own health.

You see, while traveling along the path to becoming one of the foremost physicians on the planet, Fuster had an epiphany.

He discovered that the most important predictor of the long-term well-being of his patients was their lifestyle modifications. And, if he did not advise them clearly on their prudent action steps, their lack of insight could prove deadly.

With *The Heart Manual*, Fuster puts the pieces together into a comprehensive approach to wellness that so many physicians want their patients to have. Many doctors are limited by time to offer the drab, uninspiring advice to "eat and exercise better" at the tail end of an office visit focused on reviewing a patient's new medications or diagnostic tests or even invasive procedures. Without more detail and a deeper understanding of *why* these actions are so critical, patients are generally not motivated to change their behavior. Hours are needed to adequately review the critical lifestyle issues surrounding heart disease, and Fuster pulls together the information beautifully. He helps us recognize that it is never too early or too late to make the critical changes. Along the way, all of our appropriate questions—ranging from what we should expect from the old-fashioned "check up" to the subtlety of effectively managing hypertension, high cholesterol, and high weight—are answered. *The Heart Manual* offers the ABCs of what we should do to keep our heart and brain healthy so we can obtain long-term vitality. I look forward to sharing this work with my patients.

Mehmet C. Oz, MD
Professor and Vice-Chair of Surgery
New York–Presbyterian Hospital
Columbia University
College of Physicians and Surgeons

Preface

Medicine and journalism—two very rewarding professions. Arriving at the hospital first thing in the morning with the prospect of exploring the causes of illness and helping people—all the patients you will see in the course of the day and help make their lives a little better—it's tremendously stimulating.

Arriving at the newsroom with the prospect of helping your readers be better informed so they can make choices about issues that affect them—including how to take care of their health—is a daily challenge.

All the research work being done in hospitals to understand how the heart functions, why heart attacks occur, how to prevent and treat them better, and the work being done by journalists to make society aware of these advances are equally satisfying.

And yet in spite of all these satisfactions, it is frustrating to see how the number of people who suffer heart attacks is growing. It is one of the great paradoxes of medicine today: though we have never before known so much about the heart and the arteries, and have never before had treatments as effective as the ones we have today, never have so many people died from cardiovascular disease as now. In developed countries, almost 40 percent of women and 30 percent of men die of diseases of the heart and arteries, more than the total number of deaths from all cancers. Worldwide, the figures are on the scale of a humanitarian disaster: 14 million deaths in 1990, according to data from the World Health Organization (WHO), more than malaria, tuberculosis, and AIDS combined.

These data are evidence of a failure: the failure of prevention.

Nowadays, medicine is capable of saving 90 percent of patients admitted to the emergency room with a heart attack but is unable to prevent them from having one. And unless we do something soon, the number of victims will continue to rise in the years ahead: 25 million in 2020, according to WHO forecasts.

Perhaps the most useful thing a cardiologist and health professional can do now to protect people's health is to get involved in prevention, explaining which measures are effective and which are not, how to lose weight and not put it on again, how to stop smoking and not start again, how much truth there is in the notion that wine is good for the heart—in short, to clarify all these doubts that leave so many people feeling bewildered because genuine scientific data is often mixed with humbug. And the most useful thing that a journalist specializing in science and health can do is to help the cardiologist to pass this knowledge on.

The Heart Manual is the outcome of this idea. It is structured so it can be read from start to finish as a narrative, sprinkled with examples of real but unnamed patients—we believe that for the book to be useful, it must be enjoyable to read—but its structure also allows the individual reader to start at the chapter that most interests him or her.

This is a health book that does not prohibit anything (as you will see, even a hot dog may be part of an ideal diet), which does not impose anything (because each of us is free to make whatever choices we consider best about how we live our lives), and which presents the latest scientific data about how to prevent avoidable cardiovascular disease and delay the deterioration that comes with age.

The objectives remain the same as those of the physician who arrives at the hospital and the journalist who arrives at the newsroom first thing in the morning: to ensure that the readers are as fully informed as possible about their health and to help them make their life a little better.

Valentín Fuster, MD, PhD, and Josep Corbella
January 2006

THE HEART
MANUAL

CHAPTER ONE

It's Never Too Late to Start Taking Care of Yourself

I have a patient who said to me the day she came for her first consultation:

"I went to see a dietitian, but I could not follow her advice. I joined a gym, but I only managed to go three times. And now I've come to see you."

She presented herself as a hopeless case. She was fifty-five years old and seemed convinced that her best days were gone. She was 1.66 meters tall (5'4"), weighed 84 kilograms (185 pounds), and was depressed about how she looked in the mirror. She was also depressed about not having the willpower to stick to a diet or take regular exercise. Or to quit smoking. She had tried four times and failed every time. Her self-esteem was at rock bottom. I was almost waiting for her to say: "I've come to see you, but I know that I won't be able to do what you tell me."

Hers was a typical case: the person who thinks it's too late. Who thinks that if they were unable to start exercising at thirty, when they weighed 20 kilograms (45 pounds) less? How are they going to start now?

A typical case, then, and what we doctors have learned from seeing so many patients with similar problems is that they are not lost causes. Far from it. We have any number of studies that show it's never too late to start taking care of yourself. People of all ages increase their life expectancy and improve their quality of life when they begin to look after their health.

So I said to her: "If it didn't work out with the dietitian, don't worry. We'll try getting a balanced diet later. For now the most important thing is to try to eat a little less. Be careful not to put too much on your plate or to have two courses when one will do. And if you are eating in a restaurant, remember they most often serve more than your body needs and that you don't have to eat everything they put in front of you. As for the gym, don't worry about that either: a lot of people find it hard to stick with it. But what you can do is to make the effort to walk every time you really don't need to go by car. Try to walk a little every day. And come back and see me again in three weeks, please—no more than three weeks."

An Unexpected Discovery

This woman had never had any serious heart problem. She had never been rushed to an emergency room, or hospitalized for a sudden chest pain, or been left without the power of speech by a stroke or any other cardiovascular problem. She came to see me because she was worried, not because she thought she was sick. Nevertheless, though no one had diagnosed her, and though she did not know it, she was already sick.

In the West today, almost all of us are "sick" without knowing it.

Almost all adults have atherosclerosis, a "hardening of the arteries combined with deposition of fat." It is a disease in which the arteries through which our blood circulates gradually deteriorate. It is a process that tends to be slow and can result, decades later, in a heart attack or a stroke, which is equally serious. And it is a process that in many people begins around the age of twenty, in some cases even earlier.

To find out how common atherosclerosis is among young people, a recent study examined the state of the arteries of 760 young people aged fifteen to thirty-four killed in accidents in the United States.

These young people were chosen for the study not because they were sick but, on the contrary because they were representative of the population as a whole, and it was suspected that some of them would already show signs of atherosclerosis. What no one expected, sine they were so young, was that so many of them would already have damaged arteries.

Almost 1 in 3 had an excess of bad cholesterol. Almost 1 in 6 already had hypertension. One in every 7 was obese. And 1 in 25 had already developed diabetes. This was in a group of people who were just like the young people in any U.S. city, who played baseball or basketball with their friends, were avid video game enthusiasts, liked to go to the movies or to concerts, and led perfectly normal lives without knowing that the disease was advancing in their arteries.

So, alongside the epidemic of atherosclerosis, it seems that we have an epidemic of ignorance.

This Is a Problem of Global Scope

For example, Spain, my home country, is a paradise of the Mediterranean diet, which—with its olive oil, its fresh vegetables, its fish, and its glass of wine a day—has beneficial effects for the heart. And it's true: the Mediterranean diet is excellent, not only for the heart but for health in general.

Yet when we look at the statistics, it becomes clear that Spain is following the same trend as the United States. More than 30 percent of Spanish children are overweight: almost 1 in 3. The number of adults who are not just overweight but obese is around 15 percent: 1 in 6. The data are disturbing because obesity is, in most cases, at the root of atherosclerosis: we can find atherosclerosis without obesity, in people who smoke, for example, but more rarely do we ever see obesity without atherosclerosis.

This is a problem that is not unique to Spain. In all the countries of southern Europe, where in theory it should be easy to follow the Mediterranean diet, we find the same trend. In Portugal and Greece, too, 1 in every 3 children aged four to eleven is overweight. And in Italy the percentage of overweight children stands at 36 percent, the highest in Europe, according to the European Heart Network data for 2005.

These statistics are a disaster. The U.S. study showed that atherosclerosis begins in many people around the age of twenty. And the statistics for the Mediterranean countries in recent years indicate that if we go on allowing the number of overweight children to increase year after year without doing anything to remedy the situation, we will find the problem appearing at ever younger ages.

The Four Basic Tips

As physicians, these data confront us with a contradiction. We devote almost all our working lives to trying to cure people who are already sick, but maybe the most useful thing we can do for the health of the population is to help people avoid getting sick in the first place. So, what can we doctors do to help those people who feel fine but for whom the countdown to atherosclerosis may already have started?

For a start, we can give four basic tips: watch your diet, get enough exercise, do not smoke, and see a physician when you need to. These are the four major recommendations agreed on in 2004 by the American Heart Association, the American Diabetes Society, and the American Cancer Society because these recommendations are essential to preventing not only cardiovascular disease but also diabetes and cancer.

But we have learned in recent years that it is not enough to give advice. As well as giving it, we need to ensure that as many people as possible actually follow it. And we're not doing that. Perhaps most people know what they should be doing to take care of their health, but the obesity epidemic we are seeing in the United States and other developed countries shows that we have failed to persuade them to do so.

The Death Interval

Getting people to act on the advice: this was precisely the challenge that I faced as a physician when my female patient came back to see me three weeks later.

I had told her three weeks because it marks the critical moment when a lot of patients who have been making an effort to look after themselves, who have managed to eat less and exercise more, throw in the towel. During the first three weeks, the feeling that they are doing what they should be doing is usually strong enough to keep them going, to endure another day, one day at a time.

But there comes a point, beginning in week four, where a lot of people see only the sacrifice they are making and not the benefits. And when a patient sees only sacrifice, then their plans for a healthier diet, taking regular exercise, and not smoking—though they started out with the best intentions—fail. Because the big problem is that the benefits only begin to be apparent after three months. The time that passes between those first three weeks and three months is the death interval, when many people say to themselves: "What am I making all this sacrifice for when I still weigh the same and I don't feel any better?" And many of them give up.

So I told her to come back in three weeks because that is the time when many people need a little extra motivation to keep them going. Think of it as a long distance race. You have to know that the prize is waiting at the finish line, and that you can reach it, so that you don't give up halfway when you start to get tired of running.

The woman was in better spirits than on her first visit. She was pleased at having managed to eat less and walk a little every day. Every time she left the car in the garage was another small victory. Her self-esteem had improved and she was starting to have confidence in herself and her ability to take control of her own health. This was a very significant step forward because if you do not have self-esteem and faith in yourself, it is difficult to succeed in doing things that are good for you but require effort.

"Be patient," I told her, "above all, be patient. What you're doing is not easy. Don't forget that though you may not be aware of it, your arteries may be starting to improve, and I assure you that if you continue to watch what you eat and make an effort to exercise, in less than three months you'll find you have lost weight and you really will feel better."

A Farewell to Cigarettes: Immediate Benefit

I took advantage of that visit to talk about smoking: "If you quit now," I told her, "at first you will probably not notice that you feel better. You may even think you feel worse. But stopping smoking will have almost immediate benefits for your health. In just three months, your risk of a cardiovascular accident will be so greatly reduced as to be almost what it would have been if you had never smoked. It is not easy to get through those three months, I know, but if you manage it, you will realize that in addition to preventing major health problems, you will also have improved the quality of your life."

This is something that we have seen in many studies. Smoking has an immediately harmful effect on the blood and arteries. And quitting smoking also has an immediate effect, but a beneficial one. The damage smoking does to the lungs may be long term, which is why there are sometimes cases of people developing lung cancer ten or twenty years after they stopped smoking. But the effects on the cardiovascular system are almost instant. We believe this is because smoking has a very powerful inflammatory effect on the blood and the arteries and acts as a detonator, setting off cardiovascular accidents. When you stop smoking, the dynamite is still there because the atherosclerosis is still there, but by staying off cigarettes you have a good chance of stopping the heart attack bomb from going off.

Obesity: Immediate Damage

Something similar probably happens with our diet, though this is a far more complex problem than smoking: many more substances come into play—substances that can be beneficial or harmful, depending on the amount we consume—and the data are less conclusive. Tobacco is much simpler: we know it does damage from the first cigarette. But with obesity we have also found that the damage can be quicker than we usually expect. I remember the case of a patient who changed his job and went from working eight hours a day to twelve, which is all very well if you are comfortable with it and avoid overtaxing yourself, but this patient gave up exercise, he had problems with his new boss, and in just one year he went from being slightly overweight to being obese. Three years later he suffered a heart attack.

We might wonder why this patient's atherosclerosis was so ruthless, when the condition is usually slow to evolve, often going on for several decades before resulting in a heart attack. I think the explanation is that obesity is not like a lethal weapon, a gun pointed at the heart. It acts more like a whole army because it increases what we call bad cholesterol, reduces good cholesterol, raises blood pressure, leads to diabetes—in short, it attacks the heart on many different fronts simultaneously.

And given that obesity can cause such havoc in the cardiovascular system in such a short time, we suspect that losing weight can also bring very rapid benefits in preventing cardiovascular accidents. But there have been no conclusive studies on this question, and we have no data that allow us to be as categorical as we can be with regard to smoking.

Exercise: The Gender Factor

When it comes to what is achieved with exercise, it is very different from what is achieved by stopping smoking or switching to a healthy diet. If you quit smoking, your risk of premature death drops immediately, but it will take a few weeks or a few months before you actually feel appreciably better. With exercise, however, exactly the opposite happens. The first thing you notice is how much better you feel, even before the risk of a cardiovascular accident is significantly reduced.

But when the patient is a woman, it is often more difficult to convince her to get exercise than it is in the case of a male patient. I sometimes see men who work twelve or fourteen hours a day and still find time to put on their running shoes and go out for a jog. They have the time because they have the motivation. Among women, on the other hand, this attitude is more infrequent. What we tend to find in the female population is that the women who get the most exercise are those who have the most time for it, not necessarily those who need it most.

This is a problem that we cardiologists often face. Though many people think of cardiovascular disease as mostly affecting men, the reality is that it is also the main cause of death in women. In Europe alone, more than 2 million women die each year from cardiovascular disease, amounting to 47 percent of deaths in the female population.

So, when the patient is a woman, who does not seem very motivated to keep fit, I always try to impress upon her how important it is to get some exercise, while trying to make this as easy as possible. It doesn't matter what sort of exercise you do, I say. If there is no sport that really appeals to you, start by going to Central Park and trying to walk at a brisk pace. What is important is to maintain a steady rhythm, starting with ten to fifteen minutes and aiming for at least thirty minutes at a time, at least three times a week.

For All Ages

What does not vary according to gender is that eating right and getting enough exercise is beneficial at any age. This is true for men and women alike, from age eight to eighty and beyond. There is never a point at which atherosclerosis is so advanced that it is no longer worth caring for your health. We have studies done on seniors over sixty-five, which show that when the level of bad cholesterol in the blood goes down, the risk of cardiovascular accidents and deaths goes down, too. The same is true of hypertension in elderly people. It is likely, then, that we can slow the advance of the disease at any age.

This does not mean that people can simply wait for the problems to appear before starting to take care of themselves. On the contrary, the sooner you start, the better because, as a general rule, cardiovascular disease evolves in three stages. First, the person's life is filled with what we call risk factors, such as a sedentary occupation and an unbalanced diet, which is a process that usually begins in childhood. In the second stage, the atherosclerosis spreads slowly and silently, without causing symptoms, usually between the ages of twenty and forty. Finally, the person presents serious medical problems, such as angina, a heart attack, or a stroke, usually from the age of forty-five on.

Of course, it is better to act on the risk factors in childhood than to do nothing until atherosclerosis has already appeared. And it's much better to act in the early stages of atherosclerosis than to wait until after the heart attack. But there is no point at which a person can say: "It's too late for me because I have nothing to gain." There is always something to be gained.

As in the case of a seventy-five-year-old patient who realized that he was very ill and came to see me. "I had to do something," he told me, "because I was afraid that otherwise I wouldn't live to see next year."

And the truth is that he was in pretty bad shape. He was a heavy smoker, his blood pressure was out of control, and his cholesterol levels were through the roof. Though he paid no attention to his health until very late in life, when he did start, he was really concerned and he managed to stop smoking, reduce his cholesterol, and control his blood pressure.

Four years later, during a regular visit he told me: "Doctor, I had a friend who smoked like me and ate like me and never thought about what he was doing to himself. He died last week. I think I would be where he is now if I hadn't done what you told me."

I continued visiting him for many more years—he lived until well into his nineties—and I like his story because it illustrates that it's never too late to start taking care of yourself. And also because it illustrates how much we can improve and prolong our lives if we are willing to take control of our own health.

In essence, this story is very similar to the one about that other patient who had gotten herself through the first three weeks of watching what she ate and leaving the car in the garage and going out and walking some every day. When she came back to me three months after the first visit, she had managed to get beyond the death interval and was still taking care of himself. She was smoking less, she felt good about herself, and she had begun to feel that her health was improving. That was almost five years ago. Then she went back to see the dietitian and managed to follow her advice. She rejoined the gym and managed to go more than three times. And she is still coming to see me. She has made peace with her body, she has stopped punishing it, and she has succeeded at last in feeling comfortable in it.

CHAPTER TWO

It's Never Too Soon

PREVENTION BEGINS IN CHILDHOOD

If I could go back forty years, to the 1970s, one of the things I would do differently is the way I educated my children about their health when they were little. At that time I was associate professor of Pediatrics at the Mayo Clinic in Rochester, Minnesota, and I spent a lot of my time working with children. Even now I still see a large number of children with heart disease.

I have always been interested in what happens at that age, both in order to help sick children and to help healthy children lay the foundations of good health for when they are older.

But one of the things I did not know when my own two children were young, something that I learned later when I began working with the producers of *Sesame Street*, advising them on cardiovascular health issues, is that between the ages of four and seven or so, there is a unique opportunity to educate children because at that age they already have a highly developed capacity for reasoning and are still receptive to what they hear from their parents and other adults about healthy habits.

If you wait until your children are teenagers before you start talking to them about their health, as happens in many families, above all in relation to sexuality and drugs, you find they are no longer so receptive to what you as a parent say. And if you start before the age of four, you will probably find that the children are very receptive but do not yet have a sufficiently developed capacity for reasoning.

The ideal is to start health education at an early age, but rather than reasoned argument, what works with young children is inculcating healthy habits, such as eating fruit every day or learning to switch off the TV, and leading by example—because it is absurd to expect a kid to eat an apple for dessert if his or her parents are sitting across the table wolfing down chocolate ice cream.

The great paradox is that the vast majority of children have no significant problems between five and nine years old, and most parents fail to appreciate that this is their greatest opportunity to set them on the road to a healthy life by doing something as simple as talking with them. This was what happened to me; it dawned on me that I had already missed my chance. I am not suggesting that my children now have health problems, but if I had known all this forty years ago, I would have done certain things differently.

I realized this when I started working with the *Sesame Street* production team, who have always tried to ensure that the scripts of their programs are educational. Currently, for example, they are working to prevent violent behavior and extremist attitudes, teaching children from four to seven years old to be tolerant, to accept different viewpoints, and to respect others. In the field of cardiovascular prevention, they started by deciding to have the Cookie Monster eat fruit and vegetables. *Sesame Street* teaches children that cookies are delicious, and healthy girls and boys can eat them once in a while, but fruit is delicious, too, and good guys like the Cookie Monster eat fruit every day.

From Kindergarten On

Sesame Street made this commitment to children's health because of the alarming increase in obesity in children and the avalanche of studies showing that the heart attack an adult suffers at forty-five can be traced back to health habits from childhood. We now know that a high percentage of young people already have atherosclerotic lesions in their arteries and that the more unbalanced a person's diet is and the less physical activity they engage in, the greater the risk of such injuries. We have studies showing that between 40 percent and 60 percent of cardiovascular diseases are the result of unhealthy lifestyles that people start to acquire in childhood.

We also have studies that demonstrate that if we measure the blood pressure of a group of children in a school class, for example, the ones with the highest blood pressure in childhood are more likely to become hypertensive adults. And other studies show that the more time a child spends in front of a television or computer screen, the greater the risk of developing obesity.

What all these studies are telling us is that there is a link between a person's lifestyle as a child and teenager and their health as an adult. We do not have sufficient data to know how close this relationship is. There are cases of overweight children who grow up to have normal weight, and vice versa—cases of children of normal weight who become obese adults. But as a general rule, there are relatively few cases of obese children whose weight becomes normal as they grow up, and, on the other hand, plenty of normal-weight children who go on to develop obesity.

The latter process occurs mostly in people who did not have a weight problem in childhood but already had risk factors, such as an unbalanced diet or a sedentary lifestyle.

So the most important thing parents can do to protect their children's health in the long run is to try to pass on healthy habits from a very early age. These habits range from starting to brush their teeth even before they lose their baby teeth to fastening the seat belt as soon as they get in the car, and, in the field of cardiovascular health, eating a properly balanced diet, getting regular physical exercise, and limiting how much time they spend in front of the television. Of all these habits, perhaps the most important in terms of health is a balanced diet.

Learning How to Eat

There are, however, two major problems in relation to what our children and teenagers eat. One is that their diet is often insufficiently varied, with too much sugar and saturated fat. The other problem is that they overeat: we give them too much food or we let them eat too much, and worst of all, we let them drink too much "juice" and other sweet liquids.

Children should not be pressured to finish everything they have on their plate when they no longer feel hungry. The old idea that a chubby child is a healthy child may have made some sense in the past, when many children were weak and undernourished, but nowadays infant malnutrition has all but disappeared in the developed world and instead we have the opposite problem: the overnourished child. And rather than bring children up to eat everything that is put in front of them, we should educate them in the opposite direction: not to go on eating when they're not hungry anymore.

Perhaps some parents see this as a question not of hunger but of discipline: "You'll finish it because I say so." But forcing a child to eat when he/she isn't hungry is not discipline; it's harming him/her.

Equally mistaken is the old idea that children need a different diet from adults, with plenty of meat and dairy products because they are growing. In fact, the adult body is also in permanent construction and needs to produce millions of new cells every day to replace those that die. And various studies that have looked at the diet cardiologists and health professionals recommend for adults have concluded that it is equally suitable for growing children.

So, the ideal diet for children and teenagers should be based on fruit, vegetables, cereals (preferably whole grain), fish, meat, and dairy products. Since the main sources of saturated fat in children's diets tend to be whole milk, cheese, and meat, it is advisable to opt for skimmed or semi-skimmed milk, low-fat cheese, and lean meat—or, in the case of chicken, to remove the skin. At the same time, we should not limit children's consumption of unsaturated fats such as olive oil, nuts, or fish.

This is the ideal diet we should be aiming at. The reality, however, is that we tend to stray from it. In the last twenty years we have seen a decline in the nutrition of our children and teenagers: they are consuming more soft drinks, more processed foods, and fewer home-cooked meals; more fried food and more calories and at the same time fewer nutrient-rich foods; less fruit, fewer vegetables (except potatoes, of course); lots of French fries, which has become the main food of vegetable origin; tons of salt (far more than is good for us); too much sugar, especially in preschool children; too little calcium—all in all, a disastrous state of affairs.

Now, it is not a question of banning soft drinks, factory baked goods, cake on Sundays, or candy at a birthday party. Prohibiting them would be absurd, even counterproductive because it would probably make children want them all the more. But eating doughnuts, even doughnut holes, or bags of potato chips every day is equally absurd. Perhaps we need to stop thinking of these products as food, as staples for daily consumption, and treat them as we did, not so many years ago: occasional treats alongside an otherwise balanced diet. And maybe we should also, for our children's sake, revive the custom of lunch or dinner—or breakfast, at least—as a time when the whole family eats together. When we go to the supermarket or when we prepare food at home, we could take the opportunity to talk to our children about the value of different foods. And we should set an example, with the attitude of "do as I do" rather than "do as I say," to help them acquire the habit of a healthy diet.

Learning to Be Active

If the trend in children's diet is a disaster, exercise is not much better. Physical activity has many benefits for children and teenagers. Without necessarily taking the form of competitive sports or an organized program—it may be something as simple as riding a bicycle or kicking a ball around during playtime—encouraging exercise is probably the best way we can help our children grow up healthy and happy. Playing with children encourages children's activity and moves stationary parents as well.

We know that physical activity helps control weight, that it reduces blood pressure, that it increases good cholesterol, that it enhances children's psychological well-being, that it boosts their confidence in themselves and improves their self-esteem. We also know that sedentary children tend to become sedentary adults, whereas physically active children are more likely to be physically active men and women. All of this has been demonstrated in numerous studies. The evidence that physical activity is beneficial is so irrefutable that the American Heart Association recommends that all children over four years old and all teenagers devote at least thirty minutes a day to moderate, fun activities with exercise and at least thirty minutes to intense activity at least three times a week.

But when we look at the statistics, the results are disheartening. In the United States—and the same trend is apparent in other developed countries—a survey of teenagers conducted in 2003 revealed that 30 percent of boys and 40 percent of girls had not done any kind of physical activity in the previous seven days. Not that they had done less than the recommended amount, which is less than thirty minutes a day: they had done nothing—no exercise at all in an entire week.

And when we ask ourselves why this happens, we find there are many causes, all of them very difficult to deal with. On the one hand, children and teenagers today play outdoors less often than previous generations did, and instead spend their leisure time in sedentary activities, such as watching TV or playing computer games: this is the most obvious reason. But why do children watch so much TV?

What we have here is essentially a town planning problem: in many parts of our big cities there are no play spaces large enough and safe enough for children to run around outdoors. Another problem is that children today tend to go places by car rather than on foot or by bicycle, as they would have done in the past. Then, too, we have a problem of family organization, with the increase in the number of families in which both the father and the mother work outside the home—in itself a significant social advance—and in the number of single-parent families, with children living only with their mother or their father, and this limits parents' ability to ensure that their children get enough exercise.

It would be unfair to blame children and teenagers for not getting enough exercise because it seems that everything conspires to keep them inactive. Experience shows that if they are encouraged to find some sort of exercise that they enjoy, the vast majority of children prefer to be active.

The first thing we can do at home and at school to stimulate children is to present the activity as fun, not as a competition. We are trying to produce healthy people, not champions. If there is an element of competition, it should be with oneself, in the sense of personal progress: "The better you do, the better it is for you." Children who feel pressured to win, with winning being made the primary motivation in sports, will give it up completely when they start losing or as they get older.

It is also important to help children find an activity they really enjoy. Not all children have the same likes—this seems so obvious that it's surprising how often we overlook it—and we should not make a child play tennis if they are really interested in soccer. Forcing a child to engage in a sport or activity they don't like is the worst favor we can do for them because they may end up rejecting it and, by extension, all other activities.

If a child is not particularly attracted to any one activity, the best thing usually is to let them try a variety of activities while reminding them that it need not be a sport with rules—it could be anything from Rollerblading to hiking. Basically, all children love doing some sort of physical activity.

Even those children who feel awkward and are not very coordinated, or are overweight, or have a disability, almost always end up finding a healthy activity they like. These are probably the children who benefit most from physical activity because they gain so much in self-esteem and self-confidence. So rather than saying "My child is useless at sports" and simply giving up, keep looking for alternative activities until you find one that he or she likes.

Parents must insist on gym as part of the school curriculum. More schools are adding educational classes, even to the elimination of lunch periods, to give students a "scholastic advantage." PTAs must constantly monitor this and pay attention to school boards who overly focus on scholastic activities to the detriment of gym time and lunch time.

Learning How to Watch TV

Rather than directly encouraging exercise, another effective strategy for helping children and teenagers keep physically active is to try to limit sedentary activities.

There has been a lot of research into the effects of television on children's health, and almost all of it points to the same conclusions. Less research has been done about computers because they are a more recent phenomenon, but what there is points in the same direction. The more time children spend watching TV, the more likely they are to become overweight or obese, either because they eat while they watch or because they see lots of ads for high-calorie snacks, which they then nag their parents to buy for them. In addition, all of the time they spend in front of the TV or computer is time not spent on other, generally more constructive activities like playing, reading, hanging out with their friends, or doing homework.

Another disturbing finding is that children who are left in front of the TV without adult supervision learn to accept the violence that is so prevalent in the realm of fiction without understanding the extent to which violence harms and kills real people in the real world. They can also end up believing it is right to use force to solve problems, as the good guys sometimes do in films.

This is not to say that television cannot be educational. On the contrary: it can be an excellent educational tool, as in the case of *Sesame Street* and other quality programs. The problem is that too often it has a negative effect.

In order to promote the use of TV in ways that are not detrimental to children and teenagers, the American Pediatric Association has published a set of recommendations aimed at families: these include limiting the time children spend sitting in front of the TV or computer to a maximum of an hour or two a day, not having the TV on while doing homework, not letting children have a television in their own room, and helping them choose the programs they watch. The association also recommends that adults try to watch TV with their children and teenagers whenever possible and pick up on what appears on the screen to talk about—sexuality, drugs, or violence—or about what is good and what is bad according to the values of each family, to help children understand that the ads are designed to persuade us to buy things we probably do not need, and to teach them to turn off the TV when the program they wanted to watch is over.

Learning How to Say No

Of course, it is all very well to say these things in a book: the problem is to carry the good advice over into real life and ensure that our children pay attention to what we tell them. Typically, when parents discover that their son or daughter is smoking, they try talking to them, explaining how harmful smoking is, but even after all their efforts they usually find the child still hasn't quit.

It is worth remembering here that the strategies for encouraging a youngster to lead a healthy life vary with age. In children under five the best approach is to lead by example, so that the child sees that what is normal—what is done at home—is not to smoke, to eat fruit every day, and to get out of the house on the weekend. Surveys done in nursery schools show that children whose parents smoke tend to say that smoking is okay and that they are more likely to smoke when they are older.

In some children aged four to seven years—though exact ages vary from child to child—the most effective strategy is to explain the harm that smoking and other drugs, including alcohol, do (Fig. 1), teaching them that saying no to the first puff is the best way to avoid becoming addicted to cigarettes and showing them how ads try to trick people into believing that smoking is cool. This is the time when it is most useful to talk to children in school about the human body because this is the age at which they are most receptive to health education.

But with teenagers, talking about how much harm smoking or other drugs do will have little impact. It may be too late, but it's not hopeless. Teenagers already know that cigarettes are dangerous, but the detrimental effects are so long term that they ignore them, while the short-term "rewards," such as feeling grown-up or part of a group of friends, matter more. Studies of what leads young people to start smoking indicate that the number one factor is pressure from their peers. So the best thing parents can do is to teach their children to learn to say no, even though the rest of the group is pressuring them to say yes. And remember that at this age what parents say sometimes carries less weight than the example set by people teenagers look up to as role models, such as athletes, celebrities, older siblings, or leaders of their group of friends.

figure 1

DRUGS THAT MAY CAUSE ADDICTION

● Yes ● Possibly ○ Probably not

Medicine/Drug	Psychological Dependence	Physical Dependence
Depressive/Sedative		
Alcohol	●	●
Narcotics	●	●
Sleeping pills (hypnotics)	●	●
Benzodiazepines (anxiolytics)	●	●
Inhaled substances	●	●
Volatile nitrites	●	○
Stimulants		
Amphetamine	●	●
Methamphetamine (speed)	●	●
Methylenedioxymethamphetamine (MDMA, ecstasy)	●	●
Cocaine	●	●
2-5-dimextoxy-4-methylenephetamine	●	●
Phencyclidine (PCP, angel dust)	●	●
Hallucinogens		
Lysergic Acid Diethylamide (LSD)	●	●
Marijuana	●	●
Mescaline	●	●
Psilocybin	●	●

What we are doing on *Sesame Street* at a younger age is precisely this: trying to help children learn to say no. The programs teach that smoking and taking other drugs is the soft option, and that saying no is more difficult.

We are committed to stressing this point: smoking does not make you look cool or tough—on the contrary, you show you are tough by not smoking. And the same thing is true of alcohol, marijuana, or unwanted sexual relations: the easy option is to give in to peer pressure, but the strong person is the one who, when others are trying to lead her where she does not want to go, is able to say: "I'm not going there."

CHAPTER THREE

Checkups

WHAT I SHOULD KNOW ABOUT MY HEALTH

One day a forty-two-year-old man came to see me. He played sports, followed a healthy diet, was a non-smoker; in other words, this was a man who took care of himself. However, he occasionally had palpitations, felt his heart suddenly pounding hard, and was worried because he had read that 10 percent of heart attacks hit without warning, which is true, and kill people who just the day before had thought they were perfectly healthy. He had had his blood pressure taken and it was normal; he had a blood test to check his cholesterol and that was normal, too; and he wanted to know if there was any other procedure that would tell him if his heart was healthy.

"Look, don't worry about the palpitations," I told him. "A lot of people have palpitations, and they are not a cause for concern except for a very few cases. We will check to see if you are one of those cases, but the most likely thing is that you are not."

"But is there some test that can tell me the risk of my having a heart attack?" he insisted. "Maybe a computer tomography for coronary calcium? Or a stress test?"

"Yes, there are tests. We can estimate the likelihood of a person suffering a heart attack in the next ten years using what we call the Framingham risk factor scale (Fig. 2). It is not difficult to calculate—I'll explain how it works in a moment. The risk is

figure 2

CARDIAC RISK FACTORS

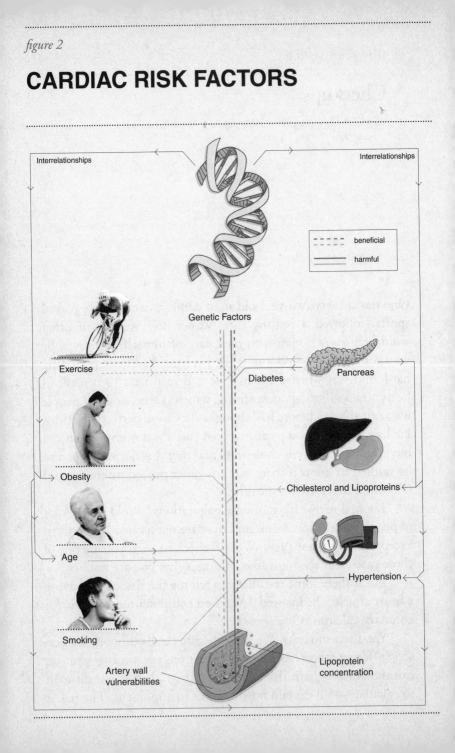

Interrelationships

Interrelationships

- - - - beneficial
———— harmful

Genetic Factors

Exercise

Diabetes   Pancreas

Obesity

Cholesterol and Lipoproteins

Age

Hypertension

Smoking

Artery wall
vulnerabilities

Lipoprotein
concentration

never zero. Not even I have zero risk, and I'm a cardiologist. But if you want an accurate assessment of your risk and want to keep that risk as low as possible, not only for cardiovascular disease but also for cancer and diabetes, the best thing is neither a computer tomography nor an effort test. The best thing is regularly to take the eight tests recommended by the American Heart Association, the American Cancer Society, and the American Diabetes Society" (Fig. 3).

These tests are a kind of wear-and-tear examination of the human body, the regular checkups we should all have done once we reach a certain age to ensure that the body does not suffer an unexpected breakdown.

Weight Control

The number one test is weight because being overweight or obese is the most important factor in the onset of diabetes and cardiovascular disorders. In fact, obese people account for three out of four cases of diabetes and half of all hypertension cases.

Now, obesity is not in itself a disease. A person can be obese and feel perfectly well, and may never suffer any serious medical condition related to their obesity. But an excess of fat in the body, particularly in the waist, sets off a cascade of biochemical reactions that, for a lot of people, ends up in an emergency room.

Medical associations recommend that from the age of twenty on we all check our weight every time we visit our family physician. For people who feel fine and only rarely see the doctor, which is most of us between twenty and forty years old, it may be enough to get on a scale once a year. That's all people with normal weight need to do.

On the other hand, if you have a tendency to put on weight easily, or are trying to lose weight, you should have a scale at home so you can weigh yourself more often. But neither is it advisable to weigh yourself every day. Getting on the scale once a week, preferably first thing in the morning and preferably naked, is sufficient.

The problem with having a scale at home is that though it is useful for controlling weight, it makes weighing yourself so easy that it can become an obsession. And, in fact, both gaining weight and losing weight are slow processes in which there is no point in weighing yourself every day. When a person gets on the scale every morning and notes a significant weight change from one day to the next, this is often due to the difference in the amount of fluid in the body, or the amount of food eaten in the last few hours, rather than the amount of fat. The only people who are really advised to weigh themselves every day are people on diuretics because they have to make sure they take the proper dosage of the drug and are not retaining or eliminating too much water. But for anyone not taking diuretics, once a week is enough.

What you need to know to find out if you are the right weight is what we call the body mass index (BMI) (Figs. 4 and 5) or see waist measurements in chapter 6.

It is not enough to get on the scale, look in the mirror and say "one hundred fifty pounds! I'm in great shape!" Because 150 pounds may be too little or too much, depending on how tall you are. The BMI is a precise indicator of whether a person's weight is right for their height.

BMI is calculated by dividing weight in kilograms (or pounds x 170) by the square of height in meters (or in inches). For example, the patient I had in my office, who weighed 70 kilograms (145 pounds) and measured 1.70 meters (5' 7"), had a BMI of 70 (or 145 x 170) divided by 2.89 (or 5 x 12 + 7), which works out at 24.2: an optimal BMI.

A BMI of below 18.5 is underweight, which can be as much a cause for concern as being overweight. Between 25 and 30 is overweight, and over 30 is obesity. Over 40 is morbid obesity. But a BMI between 18.5 and 25, the segment my patient was in, is considered to be ideal.

figure 3

ROUTINE CHECKUPS TO PREVENT CARDIOVASCULAR DISEASE AND THE MOST FREQUENT CANCERS

Review tables recommended

	20 years	30 years	40 years	50 years
Tobacco usage, exercise	Every regular medical checkup			
Blood pressure, BMI (diet)	Every regular medical checkup (or at least every 2 years if blood pressure is less than 120/80 mmHg)			
Lipidic profile	Every 5 years			
Glycemia test (glucose in the blood)			Every 3 years	
Clinical Breast Examination (CBE) and Mammogram	CBE every 3 years		Yearly CBE and Mammogram*	
Pap smear	Yearly	Every 1–3 years; depending on type of test and previous results		
Colonoscopy				Frequency depends on preferred test
Prostate and Rectal Examinations				Offered every year, helps to make informed decisions

*Some medical societies suggest less often, starting at age fifty.

figure 4

BODY MASS INDEX IN CHILDREN 2 TO 18 YEARS OLD

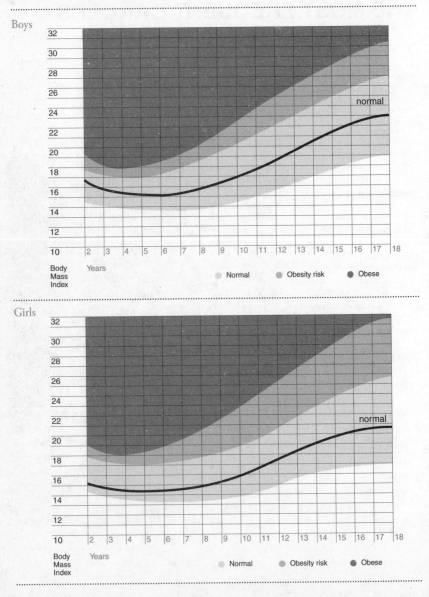

Boys

Girls

figure 5

ADULT BODY MASS INDEX

18 years or older

The Body Mass Index (BMI) is calculated using the following formula:

$$BMI = \frac{weight\ (lb)}{height^2\ (in)} \times 703$$

For example, a person who's 5'5" (5x12+5) and weighs 150 pounds would calculate their Body Mass Index as follows:

$$BMI = \frac{150}{65^2} \times 703 = 24.96$$

A BMI below 18.5 indicates underweight.

A BMI between 18.5 and 24 is ideal.

A BMI between 25 and 30 indicates overweight.

A BMI between 31 and 40 indicates obesity.

A BMI higher than 40 indicates morbid obesity.

Height	Under-weight	Ideal weight	Over-weight	Obese	Morbid obesity
58	Less than 91	91–115	119–138	143–186	More than 186
59	Less than 94	94–119	124–143	148–193	More than 193
60	Less than 97	97–123	128–148	153–199	More than 199
61	Less than 100	100–127	132–153	158–206	More than 206
62	Less than 104	104–131	136–158	164–213	More than 213
63	Less than 107	107–135	141–163	169–220	More than 220
64	Less than 110	110–140	145–169	174–227	More than 227
65	Less than 114	114–144	150–174	180–234	More than 234
66	Less than 118	118–148	155–179	186–241	More than 241
67	Less than 121	121–153	159–185	191–249	More than 249
68	Less than 125	125–158	164–190	197–256	More than 256
69	Less than 128	128–162	169–196	203–263	More than 263
70	Less than 132	132–167	174–202	209–271	More than 271
71	Less than 136	136–172	179–208	215–279	More than 279
72	Less than 140	140–177	184–213	221–287	More than 287
73	Less than 144	144–182	189–219	227–295	More than 295
74	Less than 148	148–186	194–225	233–303	More than 303
75	Less than 152	152–192	200–232	240–311	More than 311
76	Less than 156	156–197	205–238	246–320	More than 320

(The Body Mass Index Table on page 28 will show you at a glance if your weight is appropriate for your height. The values are only valid for adults, not for children and teenagers because while the body is still growing the numbers for underweight, overweight, and obese vary according to age.)

Blood Pressure

The second test everyone is recommended to take is blood pressure, which measures the pressure at which the blood circulates through their arteries. If the pressure is too low, it may mean that not enough blood reaches the brain and the person will feel dizzy or faint, especially when standing up from a sitting or lying position. If the pressure is too high—and this is a more frequent and generally more serious problem—it can damage delicate artery walls, especially in the heart, kidneys, eyes, and over time in the liver, which makes it one of the main causes of stroke.

All this happens without the person concerned realizing that they have high blood pressure, which is why hypertension is known as the silent killer. And it is no exaggeration to call it a killer: according to the World Health Organization, more than 7 million people around the world die from hypertension every year, making it the risk factor that claims most lives, ahead of smoking at 5 million victims and the 4.5 million deaths caused by high cholesterol.

This is a problem so severe and so frequent, and for many people so treacherous, that medical associations advise everyone over twenty to have their blood pressure checked at least once every two years. The maximum, what we call the systolic pressure, which corresponds to the moment when the heart contracts and expels blood under pressure, should be lower than 120 millimeters of mercury. The minimum, or diastolic pressure, which corresponds to the moment when the heart relaxes, should be lower than 80 (Fig. 7).

Occasional readings outside of these values are not necessarily serious. There are lots of situations in which a perfectly healthy person's blood pressure will be unusually high (e.g., when seeing your physician). But if the reading is exceptional, it should be taken again during the next few days.

If in doubt, you should take your blood pressure with an automatic machine once a day, several days in a row at different times. You can also do it quickly and easily at any pharmacy. If these daily readings repeatedly exceed either the 120 maximum or the 80 minimum you should go to the doctor because you probably have what we call prehypertension. And if you are consistently reading above 140 maximum or 90 minimum, the thresholds of hypertension, you should see the doctor as soon as possible because even though you may feel okay, the time bomb could explode at any moment.

We can precisely calculate the risk. If a person under the age of forty-five has a maximum of between 130 and 140, and no other risk factor such as high cholesterol or smoking, they have a 2 percent risk of suffering a cardiovascular accident within ten years. If the maximum is between 150 and 160, the risk doubles to 4 percent.

A 4 percent risk may not seem like very much, but it means that 1 in every 25 of these people who feel fine, who enjoy seemingly optimal health, and who have not yet turned forty-five will have a cardiovascular accident before they are fifty-five. And as they get older, the risk will increase. So, if at forty-five the risk was 4 percent, by fifty-five it will have gone up to 20 percent, and after sixty it will be 25 percent. This 25 percent means that 1 in 4, with no other risk factor, will suffer a cardiovascular accident caused by hypertension. And if we add two more factors, such as obesity and diabetes, the risk is up to 50 percent: 1 in 2.

The Different Types of Cholesterol

The third test that is recommended from the age of twenty on is what we call a lipid profile, a blood test that gives information about the different types of cholesterol and triglycerides.

If the results of the analysis are satisfactory, there is no need to do the test again for another five years. In cases where the cholesterol levels are not good, the patient is usually advised to eat less saturated fats—that is, less meat and dairy products—and come back for another test a few months later to see if the change of diet has been enough to lower the cholesterol to acceptable levels, or whether it is time to start treatment with medication.

The levels we regard as acceptable nowadays are a maximum of 100 milligrams per deciliter of blood (mg/dl) for LDL cholesterol, or so-called bad cholesterol, and a minimum of 50 mg/dl for HDL, or so-called good cholesterol. Ideally, the total cholesterol should not exceed 200 mg/dl.

These levels are well below what was considered acceptable just five to ten years ago, when total cholesterol of up to 240 and LDL of up to 140–160 were regarded as satisfactory. We revised such values downward after discovering that when LDL drops from 140 to 100, the risk of a cardiovascular accident is significantly reduced. In other words, we had been accepting as satisfactory cholesterol levels that were actually dangerous. And though we do not yet have the results, researchers are now trying to determine whether lowering LDL from 100 to 75 will further reduce the risk of a cardiovascular accident.

Meanwhile, pending the results of this research, many cardiologists and other health professionals believe that we will eventually set the ideal level of LDL at between 50 and 75, and total cholesterol between 150 and 175.

Another important development in the last few years is that we are now attaching less and less importance to total cholesterol and more and more to the separate analysis of the different types of cholesterol.

Many laboratories are still measuring total cholesterol because it is cheaper to do so, and they measure the different types of cholesterol separately only in cases where the total level gives cause for alarm. But total cholesterol lumps together both HDL, the so-called good cholesterol that helps prevent cardiovascular accidents, and LDL and VLDL, which contribute to causing them. And there are cases where a person has a normal total cholesterol, but their LDL is too high and their HDL too low, so that they have a high risk of heart attack. In view of this, the U.S. National Cholesterol Education program has been recommending that the different types of cholesterol be analyzed separately.

Monitoring Blood Glucose

In addition to keeping an eye on your weight, cholesterol, and blood pressure, from the age of forty-five it is important to monitor the level of glucose (a type of sugar) in the blood. The test, which is most useful when taken on an empty stomach, is what we call a blood glucose analysis.

If the results are normal (<100 mg/dl), the analysis should be repeated every three years. If they are not good, it means that the body is not regulating the level of blood sugar properly, so we are looking at a probable case of diabetes, which needs to be treated by a physician.

If we look at the figures for the United States, where diabetes affects over 5 percent of the population, more than 15 million people in total, we can see how important this test is.

Diabetes, if not properly addressed—because it is not diagnosed in time, and this is very common—leads inexorably to cardiovascular complications, kidney problems, and damage to the eyes and the nervous system.

It is estimated that 1 in 5 people with diabetes at the age of fifty-two will suffer a cardiovascular accident before they turn sixty-two, which gives an idea of how dangerous this disease is if not correctly treated. And the risk increases with age: over sixty, almost 1 in 3 will suffer a cardiovascular accident within ten years.

In order to rule out diabetes, a person's falling blood glucose level must be below 100 milligrams per deciliter (100–125 mg/dl is pre-diabetic). As with cholesterol and blood pressure, the acceptable maximum level has been lowered in recent years. When I was studying medicine, we considered normal levels of 300 for cholesterol, up to 150 for blood pressure, and 140 for blood glucose. Nowadays, if someone comes to a doctor with this profile, we immediately regard them as a high-risk patient.

Basic Health Numbers

Body Mass Index (in kg/m^2)

Underweight	18.5	Ideal weight	25	Overweight	30	Obese	40	Morbid obesity

Blood pressure (in mmHg)

Maximum	Ideal	120	Prehypertension	140	Hypertension Stage 1	160	Hypertension Stage 2	
Minimum	Ideal	80	Prehypertension	90	Hypertension Stage 1	100	Hypertension Stage 2	

Cholesterol (in mg/dl)

LDL	Good		100	Acceptable in healthy people		130	High
HDL	Low	40		Normal	50	Ideal 60	Excellent
Total			Ideal			200	High

Glycemia (in mg/dl)

Good	100	High

Fighting Cancer: Early Diagnosis

With these four tests—body mass index, blood pressure, cholesterol, and blood glucose—we can provide fairly effective protection against the risk of a cardiovascular accident, diabetes, and some cancers. But there are four other tests that medical associations specifically recommend to prevent deaths from four of the most common cancers (Fig. 3).

The best known of these tests is the breast examination. In order to detect a breast cancer in its early stages, when the chances of treating it successfully are high, it is recommended that gynecologists examine the breasts of all women over twenty once every three years. In the twenty to forty age group, breast cancers are rare, but those few that do occur tend to be virulent, so early diagnosis is vital. Over forty, when the number of cases of breast cancer starts to increase, a yearly breast examination is advisable and should be accompanied by a mammogram, also once a year.

In order to prevent cervical cancer, sexually active women aged between twenty and thirty are advised to have a yearly gynecologic cytology. From the age of thirty on, if the results of previous cytologies have been good, the test may be done every three years. Cytology detects precancerous lesions caused by human papilloma virus, which is sexually transmitted and is the origin of cervical cancer. Tests developed in the last few years, which may come to complement conventional cytology, no longer check for abnormal cells in the cervix but look directly for papilloma virus. Also developed in recent years are papillomavirus vaccines which could render cervical cancer, currently very prevalent in some regions, a residual disease. This means that the recommended steps for preventing cervical cancer are likely to change in the near future. But for the time being, sexually active women should still have a regular cytology.

In order to facilitate early diagnosis of prostate cancer, men should be informed of the relative effectiveness and limitations of the PSA test (Prostate Specific Antigen) and digital rectal examination, or DRE. The PSA test monitors the levels in the blood of a prostate-secreted protein, which scores high in cancer patients, though this may also be due simply to prostate enlargement seen with normal male aging. DRE is used to detect if there is any abnormal mass in the prostate, but neither is conclusive. With both techniques, any suspicion of a possible tumor is followed up by a biopsy, which in most cases proves normal. Given the lack of precision in both the PSA test and the DRE, medical associations recommend that all men over fifty should be offered the option of taking the tests once a year. The tests should be offered but not obligated: the individual patient, having been informed of the pros and cons of the two techniques, must decide, guided by the physician if he wants to have the tests or not.

Finally, for early diagnosis of colorectal cancer, one of the most frequent cancers in developed countries, colonoscopy is highly effective. This is an imaging technique that lets us look at the interior of the colon to see if there are polyps or tumors and to extract tissue samples for analysis. Here the results really are conclusive, and the medical associations recommend the test for both men and women over fifty. But because many people find the test unpleasant, there is no recommended frequency: how often the test is done is a question of individual choice, better guided by the physician.

Unnecessary Tests

"So, you're not advising either computer tomography or a stress test?" my patient asked.

"If you had a high risk of cardiovascular accident, I might advise such tests. But for someone like you, with no significant risk factor, they will tell us next to nothing. Unfortunately, as yet there is no test that could give you the kind of assurance you are looking for, a guarantee that you will not suffer a heart attack tomorrow. The best we can do is tell you that it is very unlikely. We can even assure you that the risk of you suffering a heart attack in the next twelve months is less than 0.1 percent, and less than 1 percent in the next ten years. But we cannot guarantee zero."

He was a well-informed patient, there is no doubt of that. Computer tomography is an imaging technique that lets us check the state of the coronary arteries in a non-invasive way: either checking the degree of calcification of the coronary arteries or looking at their narrowings after injection in a vein of contrast material without causing a great deal of discomfort. In high-risk individuals it is useful for assessing the level of atherosclerosis in the coronary arteries. To date, however, there is no evidence that the technique serves to predict the likelihood of heart attack in low-risk populations. It may be that in years to come the technique will be perfected and prove useful for people who have a low cardiovascular risk, but for now may be recommended only for high- and medium-risk patients.

Much the same is true of stress tests, which monitor the heart while the patient engages in intense physical activity. Several studies have confirmed that if the result of the stress test is abnormal, there is a greater risk of a cardiovascular accident in the future.

This is why the stress test may be recommended for high-risk subjects or men over forty-five and women over fifty-five who start doing sport after leading a sedentary life for years. The difference between men and women is because cardiovascular accidents start to occur about ten years earlier in males than in females. However, when we do the test on a low-risk individual, even if the result is abnormal, the person who leaves the doctor's office still rates as low-risk. So the test achieves little, beyond making the patient more concerned than they were before they took it.

Concerned About Your Pulse

"And what about palpitations?" my patient insisted. "If you had them, wouldn't you be worried?"

"The vast majority of palpitations are completely benign," I replied to reassure him. "A lot of people are concerned about their pulse because that is the most evident aspect of the heart's functioning, but it is of very minor importance."

Except in extreme cases within a pulse of 50 to 100 beats per minute, there is no relation between a faster or slower pulse and cardiovascular risk. Nor is it significant whether the heart takes a longer or shorter time to recover its normal rhythm after making an effort; there are athletes whose pulse rate goes up and down very quickly, and others who are slower: it has no bearing at all on health. And neither do those palpitations, when you are aware of your heart beating very hard: they are completely normal.

There are other, relatively rare cases in which an abnormal pulse is worrisome, and a visit to the doctor is advisable. A very slow pulse of less than 50 in people over sixty can cause dizziness, the feeling that one is going to pass out because not enough blood is getting to the brain, and a pacemaker implant may be recommended. A very fast pulse over 100, so called tachycardia, with no apparent cause is also worth looking into, as it may be due to what is known as atrial fibrillation. You should see your physician if you have a prolonged tachycardia and if tachycardia or palpitations are accompanied by a feeling of shortness of breath or dizziness. But apart from these exceptional cases, there is no reason to attach any great importance to the pulse.

The Framingham Verdict

Before concluding the consultation, I showed the patient a Framingham scale and explained how it worked. This is a test in which, the more points a person scores, the greater their risk of a cardiovascular accident within ten years. You do not have to be a cardiologist to use it; we have included the test on the following page to let you calculate your own level of risk.

"In your case," I told him, "an age of forty-two gives you zero points. Your total cholesterol is 175, and that gives you three points. You don't smoke, so zero points for tobacco. Your HDL, or good cholesterol, is 61, which is very high, and takes off one point. And you score zero points for absence of diabetes and for blood pressure because the maximum is under 120."

Total score: zero plus zero plus zero plus zero plus three minus one makes two points, which means that you have a low risk of suffering a cardiovascular accident, a risk of 1 percent over the next ten years. I hope this helps you feel less anxious.

How Do I Know What Risks I May Have?
Framingham Heart Study

Cardiologists use the Framingham Heart Study as a scale to calculate the approximate risk a person may have of suffering a heart attack in the following ten years. To know your risk, add the points that correspond to you in the first five tables and see the results in the final table.

Age	Points
20–34	-9
35–39	-4
40–44	0
45–49	3
50–54	6
55–59	8
60–64	10
65–69	11
70–74	12
75–79	13

Total Cholesterol (mg/dl)	Points according to age				
	20–39	40–49	50–59	60–69	70–79
<160	0	0	0	0	0
160–199	4	3	2	1	0
200–239	7	5	3	1	0
240–279	9	6	4	2	1
≥280	11	8	5	3	1

	Points according to age				
	20–39	40–49	50–59	60–69	70–79
Nonsmoker	0	0	0	0	0
Smoker	8	5	3	1	1

Cholesterol HDL (mg/dl)	Points
≥60	-1
50–59	0
40–49	1
<40	2

Diabetes	Yes	No
	4	0

Maximum Blood Pressure (mmHg)	With no treatment	With Treatment
<120	0	0
120–129	0	1
130–139	1	2
140–159	1	2
≥160	2	3

Coronary Heart Disease Risk Within the Next 10 Years	
Total Points	Risk (%)
<0	<1
0	1
1	1
2	1
3	1
4	1
5	2
6	2
7	3
8	4
9	5
10	6
11	8
12	10
13	12
14	16
15	20
16	25
≥17	≥30

Source: National Heart, Lung, and Blood Institute (USA) and the American Heart Association

How Do I Know What Risks I May Have?
Framingham Heart Study

Age	Points
20–34	-7
35–39	-3
40–44	0
45–49	3
50–54	6
55–59	8
60–64	10
65–69	12
70–74	14
75–79	16

Coronary Heart Disease Risk Within the Next 10 Years

Total Points	Risk (%)
<9	<1
9	1
10	1
11	1
12	1
13	2
14	2
15	3
16	4
17	5
18	6
19	8
20	11
21	14
22	17
23	22
24	27
≥25	≥30

Total Cholesterol (mg/dl)	Points according to age				
	20–39	40–49	50–59	60–69	70–79
<160	0	0	0	0	0
160–199	4	3	2	1	1
200–239	8	6	4	2	1
240–279	11	8	5	3	2
≥280	13	10	7	4	2

	Points according to age				
	20–39	40–49	50–59	60–69	70–79
Nonsmoker	0	0	0	0	0
Smoker	9	7	4	2	1

Cholesterol HDL (mg/dl)	Points
≥60	-1
50–59	0
40–49	1
<40	2

Diabetes	Yes	No
	4	0

Maximum Blood Pressure (mmHg)	With no treatment	With treatment
<120	0	0
120–129	1	3
130–139	2	4
140–159	3	5
≥160	4	6

Source: National Heart, Lung, and Blood Institute (USA) and the American Heart Association

CHAPTER FOUR

Your Ideal Weight

WHY IT'S SO HARD TO MAINTAIN

For many years we were very wrong about what fat does in the human body. We thought of it as a passive tissue that simply stored energy in case we happened to need it one day. We had no idea it might be doing anything more. But everything changed in 1994, when researchers at the Rockefeller University in New York found that fat cells produce leptin, a hormone that acts like a thermostat for the body's fat.

Leptin tells the brain how much fat the body has in store, so that the brain can regulate the quantity of calories we ingest and how much we burn. Of the many hormones that regulate appetite, it is one of the most important.

Since 1994 we have discovered that fat cells also produce many other substances that are vitally important when it comes to managing our current account of calories and that also regulate a number of our body functions. Today we know that, by way of these substances, fat cells maintain a permanent dialogue with many of our organs, not only the brain but also the liver, the muscles, the immune system. . . . And this explains why an excess of fat in the body has so many and such varied effects on our health.

Side Effects of Progress

If we stop to think about this new vision of fat as an active tissue, which took everyone by surprise in 1994, it is really not so surprising. The ability to store fat is vital for many animals. One that immediately comes to mind is the polar bear, which puts on dozens of kilograms during the summer in preparation for the winter. But for humans, too, managing the body's reserves of fat has been vital during hundreds of thousands of years of evolution, when food was scarce and the risk of dying of hunger was great. So it is not at all strange that fat should have evolved to play an active role and help the organism survive in periods of scarcity.

One of the prices we pay for progress is that we have inherited from our ancestors a body well adapted to food shortages but ill-suited to the affluent conditions we enjoy at present. We have to make a conscious effort to limit how much we eat because our instincts, which come from hunter-gatherers who often went hungry in the savanna or in the jungle hundreds of thousands of years ago, prompt us to eat more than we need and to eat foods that may not be good for us.

What is more, we have inherited a body well adapted to a nomadic life with a lot of physical activity but poorly adapted to the sedentary lifestyle that so many of us lead today, when we can switch channels on the TV without getting off the couch.

So the obesity epidemic we have today—and it is a full-blown epidemic—is clearly due to the fact that in the developed countries we have not yet learned to live with having more than we need. And this is a cultural problem that goes much deeper than food or the TV remote. It is also present in the compulsion to acquire things, which I see every day in New York—more cars, more clothes, more power, more shares in this or that company, more TV channels in every home—this constant urge to have more, more, more. In the end, unless you stop and think "Well, what do I really need?" you can get sucked into a headlong race to consume more and more but basically have very little.

In matters of health, this inability to stop and think what we and our bodies really need, instead of giving free rein to our appetites, is responsible for the highest obesity rates in history and an explosion of cardiovascular disease.

And the problem is not unique to New York City or the United States. Learning to live with abundance is a pending issue around the world. In Spain, where it should be easier to follow a Mediterranean diet, obesity affects 23 percent of women and 18 percent of men, meaning that roughly one in five adults is obese.

Of course, some of these cases are genetic—people who follow all the right health recommendations and still have an exorbitant body mass index—but the vast majority are due to an excessively rich diet and physical inactivity. We must be doing something terribly wrong because there have never been so many millions of people on diets as there are now and yet the incidence of obesity continues to rise all over the world.

What Is the Ideal Weight?

The best way of finding out if your weight is what it should be is to work out your body mass index (BMI) or waist measurement. As we learned in chapter 3, the BMI is calculated by dividing a person's weight in kilograms (or pounds x 170) by the square of their height in meters (or inches), and if the result is between 18.5 and 25, their weight is considered to be very satisfactory. So, for someone who is six feet tall, a weight of between 130 and 180 pounds is considered ideal.

If a person's BMI is between 25 and 30, they are overweight. Over 30 ranks as obesity, and over 40 as morbid obesity. At the opposite end of the scale, a BMI of less than 18.5 counts as underweight.

The BMI is the most straightforward way of assessing an adult's weight. It is not a perfect measure because it does not distinguish between men and women; nor does it accurately reflect what percentage of the person's weight is fat, or take into account that abdominal fat is more harmful than fat on the thighs or how muscular the person happens to be.

But it is a system with which anyone can quickly and easily calculate whether their weight is satisfactory or not. If you want to do the calculation, which is not complicated but will require a pencil and paper or a calculator, you will find a table where you can check if your weight is too high, too low, or just right in figures 4 and 5.

It is important to remember that the figures in the figure 5 are not valid for children and teenagers because a person's optimal BMI varies according to age and stage of growth as shown in figure 6. For example, the average BMI for a two-year-old is 16.5, but the figure drops to 15.5 between two and six years old and then rises again.

For adults, though, there is no doubt: a BMI above 25 is overweight, and above 30 is obesity. This is true for adults of all ages, both men and women, whether muscular or otherwise. Also, a waist measurement of more than 102 centimeters (40 inches) in men or more than 80 centimeters (31 inches) in women indicates overweight and cardiovascular risk.

Is It Okay to Be Moderately Overweight?

Of course, we are not all cut from the same pattern, and the optimal weight for a well-built person may not be the same as for someone less muscular. So, when we talk about ideal weight we do not give a single figure for the BMI but a spread that ranges from 18.5 to 25, wide enough to accommodate everybody. For a height of 1.80 meters, for example, there is a margin of 21 kilograms, from 60 to 81, within which any weight is considered satisfactory.

Within this weight range we can talk all we want about whether a person feels better, or looks better, at 62 kilograms, or

72, or 80. There is no medical basis for saying that within the ideal weight range, one weight is necessarily better than another. What is not open to debate, though, is that for a height of 1.80, overweight begins at 82 kilograms. I sometimes see patients who say: "I have such a muscular build that it's going to be difficult to get my BMI down to 25." Okay, it may be difficult, but it is not an impossible goal.

If you care about your health, it is clear that 25 is the limit above which cardiovascular risk begins. Between 25 and 30, in the overweight range, the risk is not immediate and there is no need to get obsessive. But being moderately overweight with genetic or famial predisposition can lead in the longer term to a resistance to insulin and diabetes. It is also quite common for a person who is overweight at thirty to end up being obese at fifty. So it's better to tackle the problem at the root, and try to get your BMI down below 25, than to wait for it to get worse.

Even those who believe that their natural BMI is over 25 will feel the benefit if they get it down. When a physician examines a child who, for genetic reasons, has hypercholesterolemia—that is, an excess of cholesterol in the blood—she or he does not say "that's how this boy is, it's his natural state," fold their arms, and do nothing to try to reduce the cholesterol. It's the same with a patient's BMI. We know that being overweight is a major cardiovascular risk factor, and that a child of ten who is overweight is more likely to develop hypertension or diabetes, so it is better to act at once instead of sitting back and waiting to see if they have a heart attack at forty-five.

The Impact of Obesity

The reason that being overweight or obese is so bad for our health is that fat cells secrete a whole range of substances that in excess are harmful. It has been discovered, for example, that fat cells release cytokines which alter the metabolism of cholesterol in the liver, which in turn raises the level of (bad) LDL cholesterol in the blood, pushes up the triglycerides and reduces (good) HDL cholesterol. In addition, cytokines cause constriction of the arteries and raise the blood pressure. They also interfere with the action of insulin, which increases the level of glucose in the blood and can trigger diabetes. And in a perverse effect, they tell the brain "You are hungry: eat more!" so that obesity tends to lead to more obesity.

Of course, we do not yet know all there is to know about fat. And some of what we say now may well have to be qualified or corrected in the future. But we already know that while a thin person may have 40 trillion fat cells, an obese person may have two or three times that number, more than 100 trillion fat cells in total, which are also almost twice as large as those of the skinny person and secrete more cytokines.

So, when I see a patient who has put on a lot of weight in a short time, their bad cholesterol and triglycerides will usually have increased, and so will their blood pressure, while their good cholesterol will have fallen, and a glucose analysis may well show that they just started to develop diabetes.

These effects are found above all in those obese people who have an apple-shaped silhouette, with a large accumulation of fat on the abdomen, whereas a pear-shaped silhouette, with the fat accumulated on the thighs, is less dangerous. We are not sure exactly what the difference is, but we think it is because the fat cells are different depending on which part of the body they accumulate in, and those on the abdomen are much more active in segregating harmful substances than those on the thighs. A waist measurement of more than 102 centimeters (40 inches) in men or more than 80 centimeters (31 inches) in women indicates overweight and cardiovascular risk.

Over and above the impact on heart health, obesity also increases the risk of some of the most common cancers such as colon, prostate, and breast cancer and other not so frequent cancers, such as uterine, pancreas, and ovarian cancer. It also raises the risk of complications during or after surgery. In women it can cause complications during pregnancy. It increases the risk of varicose veins, sleep apnea, and gallstones. In arthritis sufferers, it makes the pain worse. And there are psychiatric studies that link obesity to an increased risk of depression and low self-esteem.

At the same time, the positive effects of obesity are minimal. The only health problem that it appears to help prevent is osteoporosis, a disease that the bones become brittle, with an increased risk of fracture, probably because the skeleton and muscles have been strengthened by having to cope with excess weight. On the whole, the most important thing a person can do to look after their health, next to not smoking, is to avoid putting on weight.

Can I Eat Fast and Still Eat Well?

The big question, of course, is how to avoid putting on weight. Here we come up against the paradox that some people find it easy to stay thin despite eating a lot, while others tend to gain weight even if they eat little. The truth is that we do not yet understand very clearly the mechanisms that regulate body weight function. It appears that some people have more "brown" fat that burn calories as heat rather than store them as fat. In addition, the mechanisms that regulate hunger in the brain are not calibrated the same for everyone, so some people tend to feel hungry more readily than others, making it harder for them to control their appetite. In this regard, the role of leptin and other regulators of appetite is of specific research interest at this time.

Since we do not know in sufficient detail how these mechanisms work, the advice we give is of limited value. It quite often happens that advice that works well for one person will not work for another. As a general recommendation, experience indicates that in order to maintain a correct weight or get rid of excess weight, it is useful to have a structured schedule of mealtimes. It matters little whether we adopt the Mediterranean pattern, with a heavy lunch followed by a siesta, or the Anglo-Saxon pattern, with a big breakfast and a light lunch. At the end of the day the important thing is not when you ate but how much you ate, and whether your diet was balanced.

A great deal has been said here about the importance of a good breakfast, a substantial breakfast, so as not to feel hungry halfway through the morning and end up succumbing to the first hypercaloric temptation or stuffing yourself at lunchtime. In my experience, there is no one piece of advice about breakfast that is valid for everyone. If your weight is suitable and stable, I would say there is no reason to change. If you eat a light breakfast, there is no problem in staying with a light breakfast. The same if you eat a big breakfast: it is not a problem. And if you are overweight, a hearty breakfast will not help you shed pounds, though it is always better to breakfast well first thing than to breakfast badly mid-morning.

More important than how you breakfast is how you lunch. The problem here is that nowadays many people have very little time for lunch—another side effect of progress. Having not much time, they tend to eat foods high in calories to "fill the tank" as quickly as possible. And that is a mistake. You can eat fast and still eat well, but to do so you have to make sure not to put speed before the quality of the food. I personally never take more than fifteen minutes over lunch when I'm in the hospital. But having only fifteen minutes does not mean I have to opt for a three-decker sandwich dripping with mayonnaise and gobble it down at a rate of 100 calories per minute. I might have a pasta salad, or a piece of fish, or any dish without an excess of saturated fats that will fill me just as well and not cause me to put on weight.

At the other extreme, taking too long over a meal can be just as dangerous as eating in a hurry. You can lunch perfectly well in an hour: no one needs longer. And it is all very well to sit back and enjoy an after-lunch chat, but the conversation is often accompanied by a second serving of dessert, another coffee, a brandy . . . in short, more calories. We have found that heavy meals, especially if they are rich in animal fats and sugar, have an aggressive impact on the artery walls, and in people who already have significant cardiovascular risk factors, the sudden rise in triglycerides that occurs after a large meal can be enough to trigger a heart attack. Even without this disastrous outcome, which is infrequent, repetitive heavy meals can also have significant negative effects for cardiovascular health.

The fact is that if you stick to a structured pattern, instead of eating at different times every day, you have a better chance of resisting the lure of the vending machine and the pizzeria on the corner to keep you going till the next proper meal, whenever that may be. People who put on a lot of weight in a short time—and as a doctor I see them every day—are almost always people who do not have structured mealtimes.

Exercise Versus Stress and Obesity

A major contributory factor here is stress, which leads many people to use food as a self-medicated sedative. In my hospital we have a big snack vending machine that gets cleared out every day. They restock it first thing in the morning, and just a few hours later it is empty again. Not because the people who work in the hospital are undernourished but because for many of them, getting up from their desk to go and get a chocolate bar or some potato chips is an opportunity for a welcome break.

Another common reaction to stress that also contributes to putting on pounds is to stop off almost every night at a restaurant with friends after work. Or get home, raid the fridge and fix yourself a drink, with all the calories of alcohol because you have the feeling that this is the first chance to relax you have had all day. These are very human reactions to the pressures that we all endure in our daily lives. In such a highly competitive society, very few of us are able to make it through to the end of the day without accumulating some amount of stress.

But when you feel stressed, instead of turning to food or drink, I would advise doing some kind of physical exercise. This means making a break with the pattern that leads from doing nothing to putting on weight and from putting on weight to doing nothing. But if you succeed in breaking out of this vicious circle, you will find that with exercise, especially if you can schedule it for just before lunch, you end up eating not more but less. On the one hand, exercise reduces stress and the tendency to keep on eating when you are no longer hungry. On the other hand, it releases substances that inhibit appetite in the brain. These beneficial effects, combined with the calories actually burned off by exercise itself, may well be the best way to stop fat cells, about which we are learning more every day, from multiplying, increasing in size, and secreting cytokines and other harmful substances.

CHAPTER FIVE

Your Diet

HOW TO LOSE WEIGHT (AND NOT PUT IT ON AGAIN)

"I've tried everything, doctor," a patient said to me one day. "Low-carb diets, low-fat diets, for a while I was almost a vegetarian. . .sometimes on my own, sometimes with the help of a dietitian, and it always ends up the same. I manage to lose weight in the first few weeks, then put it back on in the next month or so. I really don't know what to try next."

I see a lot of patients, both men and women, who have exactly the same problem: the difficulty of slimming down to their proper weight and staying there; and some, not all, eventually find a way of doing it, which means the problem, at least for some, has a solution. I help them all, as far as I can. But in every one of these cases, solving the problem does not depend on me; it always depends on the individual.

We are not talking here about prescribing a drug or implanting a pacemaker, but about what you do with your life: the food you eat, how much exercise you get, your willpower. And one of the most common mistakes is to imagine that whether we lose weight or not depends on our diet. If we shed pounds, we say that the diet works. If we do not, we say the diet is no good. As if the diet determined what the scale says. But in reality the responsibility for what we do with our bodies is ours and ours alone. Acting as if we were not responsible is the perfect way to lose control of our health.

Diets That Do Not Work

I have spent four or five years studying different types of weight-loss diets in different patients, the different claims each one makes, how effective they are in the short term and in the long term, and in the end I am convinced that most of them are part truth, part not. I have found no sound scientific basis for the vast majority of them. They are not acceptable in terms of effectiveness.

If a new drug were shown to have the efficacy and the side effects of some of the diets on offer today, it would not be licensed for sale. We would say that the side effects were unacceptable for such a low level of effectiveness. But diets are not regulated as stringently as drugs are, and there is a whole range of options for trying to lose weight for us to pick and choose from. I say *trying to lose* weight, not *losing* weight. The most likely reason there are so many different types of diets is that they are all dubious.

One of the most surprising things I have discovered from studying diets is that entirely different strategies for losing weight end up having very similar results. With the Atkins Diet, for example, which cuts out carbohydrates but places no restrictions on fats and proteins, 7 people out of 10 are still on the diet a month after starting, but after six months the figure is down to 3 out of 10. With the Zone Diet, which allows 40 percent of calorie intake to be in the form of carbohydrates and restricts fats to a maximum of 30 percent, the result is the same: 7 out of 10 after one month, and 3 out of 10 after six months. These are just two examples, but the results are similar in every diet that has been evaluated, suggesting that the determination to persevere with the diet may be more important than the type of diet.

When we look at the effectiveness of different types of weight-loss diets in the long term, it is found that over 75 percent of people who lose weight put it all back on sooner or later. I do not know any slimming diet based on changing the balance of foods—more proteins, fewer carbohydrates, or three cheers for nuts and chocolate—that has a failure rate of less than 75 percent. Statistically, this is a disaster!

If an antibiotic failed in 75 percent of cases, I doubt if any physician would even think of prescribing it.

However, within this overwhelming failure, a minority of people do manage to lose weight and not put it back on again. And if different diets have similar success rates, perhaps the reason that some people respond better than others is not the diet but the people themselves. In other words, the important variable is not the type of diet but the kind of person. So instead of asking which diet is most effective, as we have been doing so far, maybe we should start asking why it is that some people who try to lose weight succeed and others do not.

The Basic Rule: Slowly But Surely

Losing weight is not easy, as anyone who has really tried it knows all too well. And then keeping it off is even harder.

My professional experience has taught me that when it comes to losing weight, by far the most effective way is to do it gradually. This is not a sprint; it is a long-distance race in which you have to stay motivated for months in order to keep going and reach your goal. So when an obese patient comes to me and asks me what they need to do to lose weight, I generally say: "You must lose two pounds a month, no more."

"Only two pounds?" They usually sound surprised. "My last doctor told me I had to lose twenty-five pounds as soon as possible."

We physicians have yet to agree on the best way to lose weight, but in most cases, if a person is told they have to lose weight as quickly as possible, a year later they will be right back where they started because they see themselves as incapable of doing it. So, when I have a patient who is twenty-five pounds overweight, I tell them: "You have a year to do it."

If I see that the person is emotionally strong, I might even ask them to take off just a pound a month. The slower they shed the weight, the better the results in the long run. If I see that the person is vulnerable, I may ask them to shed up to four pounds a month so that they see results almost immediately and feel motivated to keep going. But that is the very most I would ask: four pounds a month.

And I do not expect them to do anything out of the ordinary. I do not ask them to take a calculator to the grocery store to count calories or to weigh themselves every morning. On the contrary, I advise them not to.

This strategy of advising patients to lose weight gradually has proved very effective. Of course, there are quicker ways of losing weight. Every spring I see people who are anxious because the beach season is approaching and they don't like what they see in the mirror, or because they can't squeeze into that special outfit for a wedding, and they make a huge effort and get rid of ten pounds in a month. This effort will solve their problem with the bathing suit or the party dress, but it will not solve their weight problem because in the fall they will put every pound back on that they lost.

If you can convince these same people to take off ten or twelve pounds in a year—and convincing them of that is not easy because it does not solve the bathing suit problem, which they regard as urgent—in many cases you end up solving their weight problem, which is far more important.

Basically, the big difference between losing weight quickly or slowly is motivation. It's easy to stay motivated for a month with an eye on losing weight for the summer, but it's a lot tougher to stay motivated month after month for a year or two years, taking off the pounds one by one, which is what works best in the long term.

As for diets that advocate losing much weight too quickly, they can even be dangerous. Although rare, I have seen patients who have suffered a heart attack after drastic dieting and radical weight loss. They believed they were doing what was best for their health and they ended up in a hospital. We do not know what proportion of the people who follow drastic diets are affected by this problem because no proper studies have been done, and neither do we know exactly why it happens.

Personally, I think it must be because the eradication of the fat in the arteries causes microlesions inside the blood vessels, and these microlesions in turn cause blood clots that in some cases result in a heart attack. But I cannot be certain of this because no real research has been done.

What I do know is that these people who go on radical diets are treating their bodies like guinea pigs, subjecting the organism to a situation about which we know very little, and this is potentially very harmful. I would absolutely advise against it.

I would be cautious in taking drugs to lose weight. There is a long history of drugs being used to lose weight, in some cases with tragic consequences: instead of preventing heart problems, certain amphetamines, thyroid hormone, or phenfluramine actually caused them. At present we have a new generation of more advanced slimming drugs, but none of them is free of side effects if used incorrectly, so they should be taken only in very specific cases and under medical supervision.

In Search of the Root of the Problem

Once you accept that losing weight is going be a slow process, the next thing is to find out why you are overweight. This is a very important step and can determine whether the attempt to lose weight is successful or not. If you find out what makes it difficult for you to lose weight, you will see more clearly what you have to do. And the cause is not always obvious. It may be genetic, in which case we cannot get rid of the source of the problem. But it may be, as I find with most of my patients, that there are underlying emotional causes for being overweight, situations that the person often endures without being aware of the damage they are doing to their health.

I see a very wide range of such situations: problems at work, problems with partners or children, money problems . . . the whole spectrum of emotional distress that can lead a person to eat more, to drink too much, to stop taking care of themselves. So, if you have tried unsuccessfully to lose weight in the past and want to try again, the best thing you can do is sit down and think about what is wrong with your life, what it is that is preventing you from losing weight, and decide if you want to put things right or carry on as before. All of us ought to make this effort to reflect on our personal situation, stop and think about who and where we are, and try to see the relationship between our emotional state and our body mass index.

I remember one patient who, after talking about his personal situation, said to me, "Frankly, doctor, there is no chance of my losing weight. With the life I lead, working lunches, the pace of Wall Street, there is no point in even trying. I know that I ought to, but I simply can't."

His was not an easy case because instead of controlling the pace of his life, he let the city call the tune. But he was not my first Wall Street executive, and some of the others, though not all, had managed to lose weight and not put it on again.

"I think I can help you lose weight without having to renounce your way of life," I told him. "Are you willing to try?"

Practical Tips

What is really helpful for patients like this man, who are carried along by the inertia of their environment, are little strategies to cut down calorie intake and increase the amount they burn off.

Think of it like a checking account. If you put in more calories than you spend, the balance goes up. The more you spend and the less you put in, the slimmer your account gets, which is exactly what we want in cases of overweight and obesity.

The essential first step here is to want to regain control of one's life. But not everyone wants to. If a person feels reasonably okay, even though their cholesterol is through the roof and their BMI is stratospheric, they may well think that their job is the priority and their health can wait. So if they do not want to change their lifestyle, a series of little strategies can be effective in enabling them to lose weight.

"The first thing I would do if I were you," I told him, "is this: when you're in a restaurant, order two first courses or appetizers instead of a first and an entree because the first courses tend to have fewer calories than the second courses, and this is a relatively painless way of starting to lose weight. Alternatively, ask the waiter to bring you a half portion, or simply don't eat all the food on your plate—get into the habit of leaving half."

This idea shocks a lot of people because it conflicts with our culture: most of us were brought up to eat everything that is put in front of us, and if we are going to pay for it anyway, we may as well finish it. Leaving half your food on your plate seems like a waste. But most restaurants in the United States and in many other countries serve larger quantities of food than our bodies need, and eating out is one of the main causes of the current obesity epidemic. It may be a little unorthodox, but recommending that patients leave half of what they are served in restaurants has produced very satisfactory results.

"And the other piece of advice I would give you is to reduce your alcohol consumption. Alcoholic beverages contain a huge amount of calories. Bear in mind that one can of beer has almost as many calories as a steak. But don't swap the beer for a soda because you'll simply be trading calories in the form of alcohol for calories in the form of sugar. If you want to lose weight, the best thing to drink with your meals is water."

"You are not advising me to eat less fat?" He sounded surprised. And no, I did not advise that. What reducing fat intake is especially good for is lowering cholesterol rather than losing weight—unless you are consuming too much fat and that is the initial cause of your being overweight. If you want to lose weight, the important thing is to cut down on the amount of food you eat. The idea that we do the same thing to lose weight as we do to reduce cholesterol is a very common misconception.

If you have an unbalanced diet with an excess of fats, you should indeed reduce your fat intake. But if your diet is balanced, you should not change it—just eat less. Because a drastic reduction in fat amounts to an increase in carbohydrates, which can end up increasing your weight—the opposite of what you intended. On the other hand, if you cut down drastically on carbohydrates, as the Atkins Diet proposes, or like people who say "I'm not going to eat any carbs for two weeks," you may lose weight, but what happens then is that your body starts burning proteins instead of carbohydrates; in other words, it burns what it ought not to.

Nor do I advise patients to count how many calories they consume. An adult male of 180 pounds needs around 1,800 calories a day, and a woman of 140 pounds about 1,500. But these figures are statistical averages and are not valid for everyone or for every day. In practice, some people need more calories than others, and the same person may need more calories some days than others. In addition, it is difficult to work out precisely how many calories you are taking in. I, for one, do not know exactly how many calories I ingest each day. It is such a complicated calculation, and with such a wide margin of error, as to be of little value in controlling weight. What counting calories does is make people obsessed with what they eat. So I do not recommend calorie counting—it's not worth your while. Nevertheless, Weight Watchers, for example, uses a single point system—1 point = 50 calories—which may be successful for some patients, who like to be guided by detail.

In order to lose weight, it is not necessary to make any drastic cuts in your diet or to become obsessive. All that is needed is moderation, common sense, and patience because the results will not be instant. If a person is motivated to lose weight, they already have the best formula. And if they are not motivated, neither common sense nor drastic diets will work.

Long-Term Success

Besides reducing the amount of food we eat, if we want to achieve lasting results, it is advisable to get enough exercise. Of course, exercise alone will not cause us to lose much weight: people who join a gym without changing their diet rarely achieve significant weight loss, which shows that the most effective way to lose weight is not to run more but to eat less.

But to help us avoid the elevator effect, where we end up putting back all the weight we lost, exercise really is useful. This is borne out by the studies: people who combine dieting and exercising are much more successful at keeping their weight down in the long term than those who only diet.

We do not really know why this is so because in theory the number of calories burned off by exercise is not enough to explain the research results. It may in part be because the muscle tissue the body gains from physical activity burns more calories than the fat tissue that is lost, so that though you may not weigh much less, your metabolism is more efficient and therefore better at not putting on weight. There is probably also an indirect psychological factor because exercise acts as an antidote to the stress that can create a compulsive need to eat. Perhaps most important of all, including regular exercise in your daily life is a part of a general change of attitude that leads you to take better care of yourself.

It is not easy to bring about this change in attitude; in fact, it is even harder than cutting down on how much we eat or drink.

The immediate reaction of many patients on being advised to take regular exercise tends to be: "But, doctor, I don't have the time." This is just not true: we can all find time for what we feel is important. When someone says they don't have the time to do something, what they really don't have is the motivation.

I know people who have extremely busy lives, people who have virtually no free time, who nevertheless find twenty or thirty minutes every day to keep themselves physically fit and active. When Javier Pérez de Cuéllar was Secretary-General of the United Nations, he always carried with him a set of portable exercise equipment and worked out every day. Javier Solana, the European Union's High Representative for the Common Foreign and Security Policy, walks two or three miles every day, wherever he happens to be. If these people can find the time to take exercise, anyone can—if they want to.

Willing Is Able

In my experience, the people who bring down their weight by a significant amount and manage to keep it down—and I'm talking about losing twenty, forty, even sixty pounds—are almost always people who come to a point where they rethink their life. They say "I cannot go on like this" and make a radical decision, making health a priority and controlling what they eat, exercising regularly, and taking care of themselves.

This is not to say they will never again put on weight. There will be times when they go through a rough patch and may gain a few pounds. It has happened to me: times when I have been under stress, gotten less exercise, started eating badly, and gained weight. This is human. Our commitment to taking care of ourselves is often under threat from all the pressures that surround us. And there are times when the pressures are so great that we give in to them, and this can happen to any of us. But the stronger your willpower, the better you will be able to resist external pressures. And if you are quite clear that your health is the priority, even though you put on a few pounds, you will lose them again as soon as things calm down.

So the problem with the patient who said he had tried everything and always ended up putting back the weight he had lost is that though he had made a number of attempts, none of them had been serious. He had taken up diets like a hummingbird flitting from flower to flower, trying this one, then that one, making brief interludes in his life, a few months during which he would try a new diet, and then go back to his old ways. But he had never stopped to examine what it was in his life that made him put on weight, and it had never occurred to him that these intermittent diets were doing nothing to tackle the underlying problem, and that if he wanted to lose weight once and for all and not put it on again, then perhaps he needed to rethink certain aspects of his life.

CHAPTER SIX

Cholesterol

HOW TO KEEP IT UNDER CONTROL

A routine blood test showing an abnormally high cholesterol level is, for many people, the first sign that something is not right in their cardiovascular system. Often these are young people who feel fine and are not aware of any imminent danger to their health. Although there is a danger, they are correct in thinking that it is not imminent. They are not usually predisposed to make big changes in their lives: some small adjustment, all right, but no more than that.

What I do when I run into a case like this is inform the patient of the risk they run and tell them what I would do if I were in their place. I never try to impose treatment to the patient does not want, even when they have a more serious and urgent problem than a cholesterol level of 250; I never fight with them. I say:

"With a cholesterol level of 250, and taking into account that you are forty-seven years old, you have a 6 percent risk of having a heart attack or other cardiovascular accident over the next ten years. Six percent means that if there were sixteen people with your cholesterol level in this room, just sixteen people, one would suffer a cardiovascular accident. And in twenty years, it would be one out of six."

But I do not tell the patient: "You have to do this; you have to do that." I try to inform them as best I can so that they can make the right decision on how to live their life, and I respect the decision they make. I believe that patients need support and respect, not duress.

Three Types of Cholesterol

In order to make an informed decision, it is useful to know some basic facts about cholesterol. For example, we could not live without cholesterol. Although cholesterol has a bad reputation and we tend to view it as an evil, each of the billions of cells in the human body needs cholesterol to make its membrane, which is the skin of the cell.

Without cholesterol, we could not synthesize sex hormones such as estrogen and testosterone, or aldosterone, which regulates blood pressure, or build some of the basic components of the neurons in our brain. We cannot live without cholesterol, so much so that our body, especially the liver, produces most of the cholesterol it needs, and only a small portion, about 20 percent, comes from the food we eat.

The problem, then, is not that we have cholesterol; it is that the lifestyle in the West favors unhealthy levels of cholesterol.

It is also useful to know that blood tests distinguish between different types of cholesterol that act differently in the human body. In fact, all cholesterol is the same, but since it is a fat that does not dissolve in the blood, it needs a vehicle to transport it through your blood vessels. What makes one type of cholesterol different from another is the "taxi" it takes from one place to another in your body.

When you have a blood test, one of the numbers is the level of total cholesterol, which is actually the sum of three parts of your cholesterol: LDL plus HDL plus VLDL. The results are generally expressed in milligrams of cholesterol per deciliter of blood (mg/dl), although some laboratories express it in milimoles per liter (mmol/l). To convert from mmol/l to mg/dl, simply multiply by 38.6 (or simply by 40). LDL cholesterol, known as bad cholesterol, is the "taxi" that makes the outbound journey from the liver to various organs, where it repairs cell membranes and produces vital hormones. Along the way it leaves small deposits of cholesterol on the endothelium, the inner lining of the arteries. The more LDL there is in the blood, the more cholesterol gets deposited in the arteries. And the bigger these deposits are, the greater the risk that one day they will cause a heart attack. Which is why LDL is considered the lousy bad guy of the story.

HDL cholesterol makes the return trip: it collects excess bad cholesterol in the arteries and takes it back to the liver, where it is recycled or eliminated. It acts like a microscopic garbage truck that keeps the arteries clean and prevents heart attacks. Which is why it is often called good cholesterol.

As for VLDL, it transports not only cholesterol but also other passengers. We could say it is more like a minibus than a taxi. The cholesterol that hitches along with VLDL is considered irrelevant compared to the amount in LDL or HDL. The importance of VLDL is that it also carries triglycerides, another type of fat, which, like LDL cholesterol, is associated with a higher risk of heart attack.

The name HDL stands for High-Density Lipoprotein, a small amount of blood cholesterol wrapped in a denser protein shell. The opposite is true of LDL (Low-Density Lipoprotein), a higher amount of cholesterol coated in a less denser or thin layer of protein. VLDL (Very Low-Density Lipoprotein) contains triglycerides, which like cream are very light.

LDL: Weapon of Mass Destruction

Of these different types of cholesterol, the one we have studied most and best understand how to deal with is LDL, the villain. Due to its capacity to attach itself to the walls of the coronary and carotid arteries that feed the heart and brain, and to form fatty deposits (what we call an atherosclerotic plaque) that can "break" from the artery wall to the lumen and cause blood clots, LDL cholesterol is one of the most common culprits in heart attacks and strokes (Fig. 6).

In addition to forming atherosclerotic plaques, LDL acts as an instigator by directly promoting blood clotting in the large and the small arteries of the heart and brain, thus further constricting the flow of blood to the heart cells. It is, in short, a criminal of many faces.

And the heart and brain are not the only victims of LDL's evil doings. An atherosclerotic plaque can form in any artery, clogging it or causing a clot. In your legs it can cause peripheral vascular disease, which is so painful when you walk, and which is also often the prelude to a bigger cardiovascular accident.

As mentioned, in the brain high LDL can lead to a stroke, a massive, potentially fatal destruction of neurons due to a clogged artery. Or it can cause an embolism, when a clot in an artery somewhere else in the body comes loose and travels through the bloodstream to lodge in an artery in the brain, which also causes massive neuron destruction.

With a record like that, LDL has become the prime target in the fight to control cholesterol. If twenty years ago we were satisfied with measuring total cholesterol without worrying about analyzing LDL, and five to ten years ago we accepted as normal an LDL of 140–160, now that we know just what it does we recommend an LDL under 100 for anyone diagnosed with a cardiovascular condition, diabetes, or high blood pressure. For people that do not have a cardiovascular condition, it is acceptable, though not advisable, to have an LDL up to 130. A level of 130 to 160 is an early-warning signal, a wake-up call even for people with no other health problems. And over 160 is today considered an unacceptable risk for anyone, a flashing red light, a level at which you must act because you are playing Russian roulette with cholesterol.

figure 6

THE HEART ATTACK

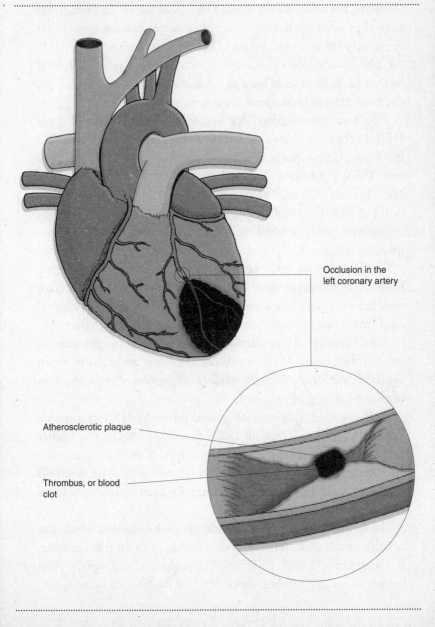

Occlusion in the
left coronary artery

Atherosclerotic plaque

Thrombus, or blood
clot

HDL: Clean-Up Brigade

About HDL, the good guy, we know less than we do about LDL. We have yet to establish a similarly clear set of recommendations, but what we have discovered in recent years suggests that HDL may be as important as LDL, or even more so.

The latest studies suggest that in assessing a person's risk of heart attack, HDL is at least as reliable an indicator as LDL. So, the two types of cholesterol are important.

We also have studies that indicate that the ratio of total HDL to cholesterol is as important as the total amount of HDL: the higher the proportion of HDL, the lower the cardiovascular risk. Thus, a person with a total cholesterol of 180 and an HDL of 60 (a ratio of 3 to 1) has a negligible risk of heart attack. But, if out of that 180 total, HDL is 36 (a ratio of 5 to 1), their risk is much higher. The ideal ratio is <4.0, and for those with heart disease <3.0.

And finally we have studies that demonstrate all the ways HDL is beneficial to our health. Most important, as we have seen before, it acts like a clean-up brigade removing bad cholesterol from your arteries. But it also has an antioxidant effect that probably reduces atherosclerosis. Wherever LDL forms an atherosclerotic plaque, HDL wards off molecules and cells that can aggravate the lesion. And it probably helps prevent the formation of stroke-causing blood clots.

In sum, if LDL is a multi-faceted criminal, HDL is a multi-faceted protector. Given all these beneficial effects, the higher the level of HDL, the better. Thus, an HDL over 60 is considered optimal, a bona fide health insurance policy. Between 40 and 60 is considered normal (average for men is 45, for women is 55). And below 40, dangerous.

In someone who has no diagnosed cardiovascular condition or other major risk factor, a level as low as 35 to 60 is acceptable. But between 30 and 35 is another early-warning signal. And below 30 we are talking about playing Russian roulette again.

If there are major risk factors such as smoking or hypertension, you have been diagnosed with a cardiovascular condition, be even more cautious and set the flashing red light to go off at 40.

How to Control Cholesterol with Diet

Bearing in mind all of the above: What is the best thing to do for that forty-seven-year-old with cholesterol hovering around 250? If this is all the information you have, total cholesterol, I would recommend taking another blood test with a full lipid profile to compare your levels of LDL, HDL, and triglycerides.

Ideally, a blood test should be taken on an empty stomach because after eating, triglycerides rise, leading to a falsely lowered lousy LDL cholesterol; HDL cholesterol may lower or stay the same. So it is best not to eat or drink anything but water for twelve hours before going in for a test.

If the results confirm a total cholesterol of around 250 (when 200 is considered high) and a dangerous level of LDL, the best advice I can give you is that you work on those aspects of your lifestyle that contribute to high LDL, starting with diet.

In some people, hypercholesterolemia, as we call high cholesterol, is genetic in origin, or the result of some other condition. In other cases, the strategy for maximum benefit with minimum risk and minimum cost is to try to lead a healthier life.

Often the first adjustment people with hypercholesterolemia need to make in terms of diet is to reduce their intake of saturated fats, found in, among other foods, beef or whole-milk dairy products. But by excessively reducing saturated fats we lower not only LDL, which is our aim, but also HDL, which is not what we want to do.

To maintain healthy levels of HDL, we must consume foods containing a type of fat that builds good cholesterol rather than bad. Olive oil, nuts, and oily fish such as salmon or sardines are rich in these healthy fats, known as unsaturated fats.

So, we face the paradox that in order to achieve a healthy level of cholesterol, we need a diet generous in fat—not in high-cholesterol foods (see below) or in saturated fats like those in red meat or milk, but poly- and monounsaturated fats such as those in certain fish and olive and plant oil. (For more complete information on fats, see chapter 10.)

To avoid such pitfalls and get guidance through the minefield of fats, it may be advisable to consult a nutritionist to help you design the right diet to control your cholesterol.

Doctor, Can I Eat Eggs?

Another common mistake is to think that in order to reduce cholesterol levels in your blood, the most important thing is to reduce cholesterol in your diet. One must reduce both cholesterol and saturated fats.

If you eat lots of high-cholesterol foods—like cheese, eggs, sausage, or crustacea (squid, shrimp)—moderating your intake of them will help reduce your blood cholesterol. In fact, doctors recommend an intake of no more than 200 milligrams of cholesterol a day, which is roughly the amount found in one egg.

But the less cholesterol you ingest, the more your body produces. And you reach a point where although you make increasingly drastic cuts in your cholesterol intake, your blood cholesterol refuses to go any lower.

Personally, I am against taking drastic measures in diet. I believe that doctors who impose severe restrictions only encourage their patients to fail, and only in exceptional cases are such measures warranted. I tell almost all my patients that they should feel free to eat whatever they like once a week: without restrictions. It is beneficial from a psychological point of view because it makes it easier for them to control what they eat the other six days of the week. And I do not believe it is harmful because your metabolism does not change overnight; it adjusts slowly to changes, and if you overindulge one day, your body deals with it easily. So when a patient asks me, "Doctor, can I eat eggs?" I tell them, "Of course you can have a celebration egg or two per week."

An egg contains all the nutrients an embryo needs to develop, and thus it is actually a very complete food. The fact that they have so much cholesterol is evidence of the enormous importance of cholesterol for living organisms.

The only thing I tell patients who love eggs is to be reasonable, and not to start each day with bacon and eggs for breakfast. But, I tell them, if they want to eat a couple of eggs a week, I do not think it will do them any harm. And if you are concerned about the large amount of cholesterol in the yolk, you can always eat just the egg white, which has no cholesterol.

Strategies for Raising Good Cholesterol

In addition to moderately reducing high-cholesterol foods and saturated fats in your diet, if high cholesterol is accompanied by overweight or obesity, as it is in most cases, you should lose weight. Not only because being overweight leads to other health problems, such as hypertension or diabetes, but because it is detrimental to cholesterol control. The higher your body mass index (several studies have shown this), the lower the HDL level and the higher the triglycerides. And a good strategy for raising HDL so that it can cleanse your arteries of those multi-offenders is to lower weight by 8 to 10 percent and, even better, aim for a BMI below 25.

Achieving this is not just a matter of lowering your total intake of calories by not only cutting the saturated fats in your diet but by also cutting the carbohydrates—particularly in sugar—and alcohol. At the same time, if you are a smoker, quitting can raise your HDL by about 10 percent.

But the best thing you can do for your HDL is to get regular exercise. Aerobic exercises like running or swimming can raise HDL by about 5 percent. And you do not need to spend your life in the gym to enjoy the benefits. What counts is not how hard you sweat but how often and how long you exercise. Fast walking can be enough to raise HDL, but in order to get the most out of it you should walk at least thirty minutes at least three times a week. And if you exercise five days a week, even better. It seems that to get the maximum benefit from physical exercise, it is better to do five half-hour sessions rather than three one-hour sessions.

When You Need Drugs

After eight weeks following these recommendations, it is time for another blood test to see how your cholesterol levels are doing. As a general rule, it usually takes two to three weeks for cholesterol to start to fall after you adjust your diet, and eight weeks is enough time to see the maximum results.

If your cholesterol is not down enough, you should complement the changes you made in your diet and exercise with soluble fiber supplements, and give it another six weeks before having your blood tested again. Fiber helps inhibit fat absorption in the digestive system and makes you feel satiated, so it helps reduce both the amount of saturated fat going into your blood and the amount of calories you ingest.

The basic idea is that diet and physical exercise are the first line of treatment to correct worrisome LDL- and HDL-cholesterol levels. Over time, adopting healthy habits can reduce total cholesterol by 10–40 mg/dl.

But for many people these measures are not enough, either because their initial cholesterol level was extremely high or because their cholesterol is not due to unhealthy, correctable habits but to their genetic makeup. In other cases, people simply do not follow their doctors' advice. There is also a large group of patients who have a cardiovascular condition and for whom aggressive treatment to reduce cholesterol is advisable.

For all these people we now have highly effective drugs against LDL cholesterol. These drugs are not a substitute for recommended diet and physical exercise but rather a complement to them. The most important anti-cholesterol drugs are statins, which inhibit cholesterol production in the liver, thereby reducing the amount of LDL in your blood. Less LDL in your blood allows fatty deposits on the walls of your arteries to dissolve and reduces significantly the risk of heart attack. Statins are also effective anticoagulants and anti-inflammatories, which further reduce the risk of cardiovascular accident.

Today, statins are recommended for all patients diagnosed with a cardiovascular condition and LDL over 130, for all people with two or more risk factors and LDL above 160, and for anyone with LDL above 190, even if there are no other risk factors.

But cardiologists are engaged in debate over whether these levels are still too high. It has been shown that the risk of cardiovascular accident drops significantly when we cut LDL from 130 to 100, and that risk continues to diminish down to 70. We do not know yet at what level of LDL the risk is minimum because there are not enough studies of levels below 70. But an evolving opinion is that in the near future we will be prescribing statins for far more people than we do now, starting with all patients that have been diagnosed with a heart attack or stroke, even if their LDL is below 100.

As it stands, only a minority of the people that should be taking statins actually take them. In the U.S., for example, only 1 in 3 people who meet the prescription criteria for statins take them. On the world level, out of the 200 million people who should take statins, the ratio is 1 in 8, or 25 million.

The data we have from Spain is no better. According to a study in the provinces of Madrid, Castile-Leon, and Galicia, 7 out of 10 people over sixty-five years of age suffer hypercholesterolemia. Among those affected, only 1 in 3 is aware they have high cholesterol. And among those who know, only 1 in 3 is being treated with drugs. And the fact that they are older than sixty-five years does not justify not providing treatment: in this age group reducing cholesterol to acceptable levels as a lifelong endeavor significantly increases life expectancy.

So when I have a patient who is worried because he just discovered that his cholesterol is 250, instead of telling him he has a problem, I prefer to make him see there is a solution. To some patients I might even say:

"Two hundred fifty? Congratulations, you're a lucky man!"

"Lucky? What do you mean lucky?"

"Yes, you're lucky because the vast majority of the people in your situation do not know they have a cholesterol problem and do nothing to treat it. But you are part of the fortunate minority who do know and can take steps to avoid having a heart attack one day."

CHAPTER SEVEN

Hypertension

THE SILENT KILLER

Having explained in the previous chapter the perils of too much cholesterol, we should now recall that almost half of all heart attack victims have normal cholesterol. And this happens because cardiovascular disease is, in most cases, the final outcome of the manifold attacks to which the human body is subjected over the years. If it is not cholesterol, it is tobacco, hypertension, abdominal fat with its toxic cytokine products, even air pollution. And after holding out for twenty, thirty, forty years, there comes a time when the body can take no more and gives up: time to call an ambulance for an express trip to the emergency room.

Among all these threats, a most dangerous one is hypertension. Yet, although the World Health Organization stresses that high blood pressure is the deadliest risk, causing seven million deaths annually worldwide, neither doctors nor patients accord hypertension the importance it deserves. Doctors because in many cases they still accept as normal blood pressure levels that, with all we know today about the human body, are absolutely unacceptable. And patients because hypertension rarely interferes with their daily lives; it seldom causes discomfort, which is why it is called the silent killer. It is a sneaky disease that does not give itself away with obvious symptoms, so most people with high blood pressure see no reason to go to the doctor.

The result is that hypertension is often poorly diagnosed, and when diagnosed, it is not always treated correctly. In Spain, for instance, 35 percent of all adults, or about ten million people, suffer high blood pressure. Those are huge figures. Among those ten million, 1 out of 3 is not even aware that they are hypertensive. And among those who do know, most do not do enough and some do nothing at all. The upshot, according to a number of Hypertension Societies, is that only 15 percent of hypertensive persons receive the correct medical treatment—only 15 percent for a disease that is one of the biggest causes of death.

How Blood Pressure Is Regulated

Blood pressure, or arterial tension, is the pressure at which the blood flows through the arteries. Or, to put it another way, the pressure your blood exerts on the walls of your arteries. To understand why too much or too little pressure is harmful, and what to do to control it, you should know that when your doctor takes your blood pressure, there are two values, maximum and minimum, expressed by two numbers separated by a slash. For example, 130/90 millimeters of mercury (mmHg) means a maximum of 130 and a minimum of 90. When the heart relaxes between beats. It is sometimes also expressed as 13/9 rather than 130/90; the same value divided by 10 to mean exactly the same thing (mmHg). The values are expressed in millimeters of mercury representing the height to which a column of mercury would rise if it were under the same pressure as in the artery. The maximum, what we call systolic pressure, is the moment when the heart contracts and expels blood under pressure. The minimum, or diastolic, corresponds to the moment when the heart relaxes between contractions.

However, it is not only the heart that determines blood pressure. More important than the heart is the state of peripheral blood vessels, such as the arteries that feed the leg muscles or the viscera in the abdomen. When the arteries dilate, blood flows under low pressure. But when the arteries contract, the pressure rises. It is like water in a hose: the more you constrict the hose, the higher the water pressure behind the constriction.

This regulatory role of peripheral blood vessels is why older people have higher blood pressure than young adults: with age, blood vessels gradually lose their ability to dilate. It is estimated that over the age of fifty, blood pressure rises 5 millimeters of mercury per decade so that for a fifty-year-old with a maximum of 130, by the time they are sixty that will have risen to 135 and to 140 by age seventy. This does not imply that we should accept such increases in blood pressure values. In fact, that is why we find that 2 out of 3 people over sixty are hypertensive.

It is also the peripheral blood vessels that explain why alcohol, smoking, coffee, and stress raise blood pressure: they are all powerful vasoconstrictors, which means they narrow the arteries and force the blood to flow under higher pressure.

Finally, the kidneys, which after the heart and peripheral vessels are the third major regulator of blood pressure, control the volume of water in the blood. The more water flowing through the hose, the higher the pressure. So, when there is too much water, the kidneys remove it in the form of urine. And vice versa: when there is too little water in the blood, an internal drought, the kidneys retain it. Here is where salt comes in, which by retaining water increases the volume of blood and raises arterial blood pressure. Which is why one of the first recommendations for people with hypertension is to avoid salt.

The Risks of High Blood Pressure

Fortunately, the human body has very precise and sophisticated blood pressure control mechanisms to deal with any given situation. While you sleep, for example, the walls of your blood vessels relax and pressure is at its lowest. When you get up, the blood vessels in your legs and abdomen quickly contract, thus raising pressure to ensure your brain and heart are not deprived of blood. When you exercise, the vessels also contract to supply your muscles with more oxygen.

But these mechanisms, despite all their sophistication, are not perfect and cannot prevent pressure from occasionally rising to dangerous levels. In these cases, the blood flowing under high pressure gradually causes the delicate artery walls, what we call the endothelium, to deteriorate thus promoting atherosclerosis throughout the circulatory system, from your head to your feet, and this can have devastating effects on particularly sensitive organs such as the brain, heart, kidneys, or eyes. In the brain, for example, blood pressure can damage small blood vessels and cause injuries that on their own are not very important but that one after another, over the years, end up wreaking havoc, leading to senile dementia.

High blood pressure can also cause medium-sized vessels to rupture and thus trigger a massive hemorrhagic stroke. It can erode artery walls where fat accumulates in plaques and cause clots that can lead to an ischemic stroke. Or it can dislodge a clot in the carotid arteries, the two major arteries running up on either side of the neck, and if the clot reaches the brain and gets stuck in a small artery, it can also cause an ischemic stroke. (See page 247 for an illustration explaining the different types of stroke.)

Similarly, for the heart, the rupture of a small plaque on the wall of an artery by the mechanical action of blood flowing under high pressure can obstruct a coronary artery and cause a heart attack. And if it does not lead to a heart attack, hypertension in any case forces the heart to overexert itself since it must pump blood harder to overcome the resistance of peripheral blood vessels, a situation that may end up degenerating into cardiac insufficiency—in other words, an inability to pump blood efficiently.

Thus, in hypertension, we face a formidable enemy whose attacks come on many fronts, and that can just as easily launch a lightning strike and knock the heart out as it can operate under the radar evading detection for years, causing gradual damage that ultimately will end up doing irreparable harm to your brain, or heart, or elsewhere in the body such as in the kidneys or the retina.

High Blood Pressure, Low Blood Pressure

All of this is hardly news. Much of the destruction wrought by high blood pressure was already known when I was still in medical school in the sixties. It is hardly news, and yet today we still shrug off alarmingly high levels of blood pressure. When someone tells me, and I have heard this many times, "My blood pressure is 150/90, but they told me it's normal for my age and I needn't do anything about it," I always tell them that such numbers are intolerably high and that they should bring them down to 130/85. I tell them that being sixty-five or seventy years old is no reason not to act because the years they still have to live, which may be many, are worth living in the best of health.

Today we believe that a maximum exceeding 140 or a minimum higher than 90 indicates hypertension and warrants changes in lifestyle, especially diet, and treatment with drugs. When the maximum is between 120 and 140 or the minimum between 80 and 90 we call it prehypertension. This means that the person does not have hypertension, but they will in the future unless they correct unhealthy habits. At this level, treatment with drugs is not justified, but improving diet, losing weight, and exercising regularly are recommended. Below 130/85 is considered normal (Fig. 7). In diabetics because of high risk, it has been suggested even readings below 125/80 mmHg, if such low values can be tolerated.

figure 7

BLOOD PRESSURE

Category	Systolic Blood Pressure	Diastolic Blood Pressure
Normal Blood Pressure	**120 mmHg or less**	**80 mmHg or less**
Prehypertension*	**121–139**	**81–89**
Level 1 Hypertension (mild)	**140–159**	**90–99**
Level 2 Hypertension (moderate)	**160–179**	**100–109**
Level 3 Hypertension (serious)	**180–209**	**110–119**
Level 4 Hypertension (very serious)	**210 or higher**	**120 or higher**

*Some cardiovascular societies consider such prehypertension values as normal blood pressure since lower blood pressures may occasionally be associated with lightheadedness (i.e., in the elderly, etc.).

These values might seem overly strict because, as such, most of the adult population has high blood pressure. But they have been established because cardiovascular risk rises from 115/75, doubling for each increment of 20 in the maximum and 10 in the minimum. So, with blood pressure of 135/85, a value that does not qualify as hypertension, the risk of suffering a stroke or heart attack is twice that of 115/75. And at 155/95, the risk is fourfold.

Of the two values, maximum and minimum, the former is usually considered more important, the reason being that the maximum corresponds to the moment when the heart pumps blood out with the greatest force and thus is usually associated with stroke, which is often the most severe consequence of hypertension. The maximum is also mostly associated with the mechanical damage that hypertension causes to arteries.

The minimum, however, cannot be disregarded because it corresponds to the moment when the heart relaxes and thus when the most blood enters the coronary arteries. So too high a minimum can also contribute to a myocardial infarction, or heart attack.

On the other hand, if your blood pressure is too low, that can also be a problem. Low blood pressure makes some people feel so dizzy when they stand up that they fall. What happens in these cases, which are more common in women than in men, is that the body takes longer than normal to adjust to the upright position and for a few seconds not enough blood reaches the brain. Typically this occurs in summer, when the heat dilates blood vessels and blood tends to accumulate in the lower body, or after a copious meal, when the digestive system "steals" blood from the brain.

Compared with hypertension, low blood pressure is a minor problem. But there is a group of people, especially elderly people with relatively low pressure, a slow pulse, and propensity to dizziness or falling, for whom a visit to the doctor is justified. In other cases, it is usually enough to drink plenty of liquids and add a little more salt to the diet in order to raise blood pressure and correct the problem.

It Can Happen to Anyone

Returning to high blood pressure, a problem that is both more frequent and more serious than low blood pressure, there is no typical profile of a hypertensive person. It is something that can happen to anyone. Contrary to a widely held belief, it does not depend on temperament. When doctors talk about blood pressure, we mean the pressure at which blood circulates through the arteries, which is independent of the pressure or stress to which a person is subjected. And what we see in the medical world is that even the most serene and calm person in the world can suffer hypertension. Likewise, the most temperamental people often have normal blood pressure.

It is true that when one is in a situation of acute stress, blood pressure tends to rise. This happens because stress causes the release of adrenaline and other vasoconstrictive hormones that raise blood pressure. But this rise is transitory and generally inconsequential. In fact, blood pressure fluctuates widely over the day, and even a healthy person will at times have maximums exceeding 160 and minimums above 110. These values, if they occur on an occasional basis, are perfectly normal and do not mean that a person has hypertension. They are no reason for concern.

We speak of hypertension only when blood pressure remains constantly high. But how to detect it, if there is often no alarm bell to warn you of a blood pressure problem? In some people, but not many, hypertension is accompanied by headache in the forehead or the temples. But there are many cases of headaches that have nothing to do with hypertension, and many cases of hypertension that are not accompanied by headache. In the end, there is only one reliable way of knowing if your blood pressure is normal or is not: check it.

To detect hypertension before it causes serious damage in the arteries, the American Heart Association recommends that all adults check their blood pressure at least once every two years from twenty years of age. In children with obesity or a family history of hypertension—a hypertensive parent or sibling, for instance—I suggest, although it's not an official recommendation, starting to check blood pressure after the age of ten.

Since blood pressure fluctuates, when in doubt as to whether you are hypertensive or not, check it more frequently (i.e., with an automatic blood pressure machine) to ensure a more reliable reading: ideally, once daily, and at different hours every day over a period of three weeks. Better yet, take your pressure twice with a two-minute interval, then discard the first result and keep the second. What you achieve with so many measurements is a good overview free from the distortions caused by natural fluctuations in blood pressure. This same strategy of measuring blood pressure once daily for three weeks is also useful when a patient first starts taking an anti-hypertension drug in order to ensure that they are responding to the treatment and that the dose is appropriate.

A Diet for Hypertension

If, after following the above approach, hypertension is confirmed, urgent action is needed. The most common approach is to reduce salt consumption. According to popular wisdom, you should try to cook without salt, keep the saltshaker away from the dinner table, and use other seasonings to flavor your food.

The problem is that it is impossible to know always how much salt your food contains and thus whether it exceeds the recommended limit, 6 grams daily, equivalent to a teaspoon of salt for the whole day. There is no way of knowing how much salt there is in processed foods from the supermarket or dishes served in restaurants. Baked ham, for example, although it does not taste salty, often contains more sodium than the cured variety. Milk, although you would hardly guess by the taste either, also contains a significant amount of sodium. Sodium is the key because it's the element in salt that causes blood pressure to rise. Pre-prepared meals, as well as some brand-name crackers and breads, are also often high in salt.

In the end, the only general recommendations one can give for limiting salt intake are to avoid processed foods and opt for natural ones instead, check food labels for sodium content, and when you eat at home, try to cook without salt and keep the saltshaker out of reach while eating.

There is a minority of people who are very sensitive to salt and in whom these measures can achieve a dramatic reduction in blood pressure. But in most hypertensive persons, restrictions on salt, while desirable, have a limited impact.

As important as restricting salt is to reduce weight. Indeed, blood pressure rises with body mass index, and in cases of over-weight or obesity, weight loss is the most effective measure for lowering blood pressure. It is estimated that maximum blood pressure can be reduced by 20 mm or even more, and cardiovascular risk related to hypertension cut by nearly half, for every 10 kilograms (22 pounds) an obese person loses.

In addition to limiting calories to lose weight, correcting imbalances in your diet is also helpful in controlling blood pressure. Of the various scientifically based diets for hypertensive people, the one that has proved most effective is DASH (Dietary Approach to Stop Hypertension). DASH is rich (i.e., 2 daily servings of fat-free dairy products); it includes fruits, vegetables, whole grains, poultry, fish, and nuts, and is low in fat, red meat, sugars, and alcohol. On average, in hypertensive people this sort of diet reduces maximum pressure by 11 mm and the minimum by 5.5.

This does not mean that DASH forbids red meat or alcohol, small amounts of which are permitted. In the case of alcohol, for example, men are not discouraged from having up to two glasses of wine or two beers a day; for women it is one glass of wine or beer, although recent studies have suggested even these amounts may be too high. Above those intakes, however, the harm definitely outweighs any benefits.

On the one hand because alcoholic beverages contain an enormous amount of calories, they contribute to obesity. On the other hand, although alcohol dilates superficial blood vessels (which is why some people's cheeks turn red when they drink), in deeper arteries it has a vasoconstrictive action that raises blood pressure.

Caffeine, in contrast, is much less important. It may seem that coffee, being a stimulant, would raise blood pressure. But no study has conclusively linked higher or lower coffee consumption with higher or lower blood pressure, and the dietary recommendations of the American Heart Association for the prevention and treatment of hypertension, which are very clear about limiting fats, sugar, or alcohol, do not mention coffee. So if a hypertensive person feels like having a cup of coffee for breakfast, there is no reason to advise against it. I would say not to have six a day—that much caffeine can hurt anyone—but I do not believe that one or two a day has a major impact on blood pressure.

Apart from watching your diet and weight, physical exercise has also been shown to be highly effective in controlling blood pressure—which may seem ironic, since, when you exercise, you make your heart work harder, which in turn raises your blood pressure. But with exercise, blood pressure ultimately stabilizes at a lower level.

Studies with hypertensive volunteers have shown that the best exercises for reducing blood pressure—as well as cholesterol—are aerobic exercises such as running or swimming, and that to make a significant improvement you should exercise at least thirty minutes a day three times a week. For people who feel stressed, taking up relaxation techniques such as yoga has also been shown to be beneficial.

Treatment with Drugs

But all these measures are sometimes not enough to reduce blood pressure to safe levels and we must resort to drugs.

There are three main types of drugs that act in different ways, and many patients need to take more than one in order to control their blood pressure. The first option is diuretics, which act by removing excess fluid from the blood and are the most effective in controlling blood pressure, but they are not suitable for all patients because they make you urinate frequently.

Then there are vasodilators, which reduce blood pressures by expanding blood vessels. There are many different types of vasodilators, and doctors today prescribe them frequently, although they have the disadvantage that they often cause significant fluctuations in blood pressure over the course of the day, as compared with the more consistent effects of diuretics.

Finally, there are beta-blockers, which reduce blood pressure by inhibiting nerve impulses in the brain to the heart and blood vessels, so that the heart beats more slowly and less hard. But not infrequently they can cause fatigue, impotence, and affect your capacity for work.

Some patients are tempted, when prescribed drugs, to stop worrying about their diet, weight, and exercise. They think, I tried, but it didn't work, and now that they're giving me drugs—why should I keep trying? They are wrong. I would tell such patients that their efforts did work, just not enough, and they need a little extra help, a small dose of drugs, to lower their blood pressure to where we can feel safe. But if you lower your guard with diet, weight control, and exercise, a little help will no longer be enough; you will need larger doses of drugs and the results will certainly be worse.

CHAPTER EIGHT

Coagulation

A STORM IN A BLOOD VESSEL

In cities, each time there is a spike in air pollution, with high levels of pollutants that persist for hours or days, there may be a spike in the number of deaths from heart failure. The victims are almost always people whose health is already fragile, who already have some pulmonary or cardiovascular condition and have reached a point where they cannot survive another blow to their cardiovascular system.

The death toll appears to be high: a study in France, Austria, and Switzerland estimated that in these three countries alone, air pollution may cause forty thousand deaths a year. In Holland, another study concluded that air pollution causes twice as many deaths as road accidents. One wonders, how is it possible? How do you explain that air pollution, something we are so used to living with, can cause so many deaths?

Part of the answer, as we have discovered in recent years, is that some airborne particles are small enough to stow away in the oxygen that the lungs pass into the blood, and once they start traveling around the cardiovascular system, they trigger a reaction with devastating effects.

The reaction is inflammation. Inflammation has an impact we had never suspected in cardiovascular accidents. And it's not just the inflammatory reaction to air pollutants, but much more important to tobacco residue in the blood, to cytokines secreted by fat, and to LDL cholesterol.

All these blows to the system encourage an inflammatory response that foments blood clotting. Whenever a heart attack occurs, that's the sign of an inflammatory reaction out of control.

What We Mean by Inflammation

We often use the word *inflammation* as a synonym for *swelling*. When, for example, you have a cut and bacteria gets into it, the immune system dispatches troops of white blood cells, mainly the so-called neutrophils, to take on the bacteria which is recognized as a "foreign" element in the body. In the brief chemical war that rages within a space of a few cubic millimeters, neutrophils release substances that halt the advance of bacteria and cause painful swelling.

Inflammation of the inner wall of an artery is very similar to inflammation of the skin, but with two differences. One is that arteries have no pain receptors to send the brain a signal that something is not right (pain, after all, is a biological fault-finder system). So we do not realize that we have inflamed arteries and that atherosclerosis is advancing.

The other difference is that what causes inflammation in the artery wall is not an infection or an insect bite but rather some substance in the blood, like your own LDL cholesterol. The more cholesterol that accumulates in the artery, as a "foreign" element, the more immune system cells come to remove it. In fact, when we speak of inflammation in the artery, we are speaking not about swelling but about this activation in the immune system of white blood cells, mainly the so-called monocytes.

Aside from the inflammation in the artery wall, there are some cases where the monocytes can be activated in the blood itself, where the toxins from tobacco, or LDL cholesterol, or excess glucose in diabetic people, attract the immunogenic troops, which launch a sometimes catastrophic attack. This is what we call blood inflammation.

From Inflammation to Heart Attack

Inflammation, then, originates in a natural defense system against bacteria, toxins, and other aggressors. But when your coronary arteries are already in bad shape, the last thing you want is to have them hosting a pitched battle between immune cells and LDL cholesterol. However, this is exactly what happens: the extreme use of force by the immune system triggers a heart attack.

Specifically, monocytes, in their eagerness to wipe out LDL cholesterol or a "foreign" element in the artery, cause cholesterol plaques on artery walls to rupture and thus there is a sudden release of cholesterol inside the artery, the conduit through which blood flows. At the same time, immunogenic troops open fire on proteins that cause clotting in the artery wall and in the blood itself.

Clotting, in another time and place, would be the correct action to heal the wound. It is the tool that the immune system uses to avoid unnecessary bloodshed. But here, in the middle of a biochemical storm inside a coronary artery, the clot tends to be excessive, obstructs the artery, and blocks the flow of blood to part of the heart. If blood fails to reach the heart, so does oxygen, and the heart is literally suffocated. Here we have the beginning of a heart attack: the death of a portion of heart muscle due to lack of oxygen (Fig. 6).

What actually happens is that monocytes (which normally do a wonderful job of removing LDL cholesterol from the artery wall and the blood itself), finding themselves overwhelmed, self-destruct and release a lethal cocktail of substances that destroy the fabric of the artery and favor the formation of a clot.

The Four Horsemen of Inflammation and Clotting

Without going as far as a heart attack, a situation of chronic inflammation can also arise where the immune system is permanently activated, continuously releasing oxidizing substances that accelerate the advance of atherosclerosis.

This is the situation that occurs, for example, in obese people, since fat cells release substances that inflame both the artery wall and the blood. It also happens in people with diabetes because excess blood sugar stimulates an immune reaction. And it occurs in people with high LDL cholesterol because, as mentioned, too much LDL also activates the immune system in artery walls and the blood. These three offenders—obesity, diabetes, and LDL cholesterol—can cause both a reaction of chronic inflammation that advances atherosclerosis in the long term and an immediate acute inflammation that triggers a heart attack.

There is a fourth offender—tobacco—but it seems to cause only acute inflammation. That is why when a person quits smoking their cardiovascular risk soon returns to a level nearly as low as if they had never smoked because the long-term damage caused by tobacco in the blood and arteries is minor. The immediate damage, however, is enormous.

As far as we know today, and we still do not know everything, smoking activates the monocytes in the immune system, which, finding themselves overwhelmed, self-destruct releasing a lethal cocktail of substances that promote clotting. It is true that you can smoke for decades without any major clots forming because the blood maintains a tricky balance between proteins that promote clotting and proteins that inhibit it. But the more cigarettes you smoke, the greater the chances of coagulation, and the greater the likelihood of the balance eventually breaking down and thus forming a fatal clot.

Flu and Other Infections

Next comes a long list of candidates to join the four horsemen of inflammation. All of them cause inflammatory reactions and all increase the risk of cardiovascular accident, but it is not always clear that inflammation is the cause of the accident. We enter, thus, the realm of hypothesis.

Every cardiologist has had a patient that having just recovered from the flu, for example, suffers a heart attack. We do a coronary angiography to examine the condition of the coronary arteries and we find just one problem artery: the one that is blocked. All the others look normal in the image.

If we had done the same angiogram on the patient a week before, the day before they got the flu, we would never have guessed they were about to have a heart attack. And yet, there they lie in intensive care. What happened over those seven days?

We sometimes call such a patient's condition decompensation. They had some previous disease, in most cases chronic, which remained stable but, as a result of the flu, something in their body was thrown out of kilter and everything broke down. Okay, but what became unbalanced and how?

In some cases, flu can lead to myocarditis, for example, an inflammation of the muscular part of the heart. But in others, a leading hypothesis is that flu triggers an activation of the immune system, which in turn causes blood inflammation of the blood and (or) arterial wall, which eventually leads to heart attack. In the vast majority of infections, this domino effect ending up in a heart attack goes unseen. If you have hepatitis, or herpes, or gastroenteritis, there is no reason to fear that your heart might be in danger. But there are other infections, besides the flu, where there seems to be a relationship with cardiovascular risk.

Several studies have targeted *Chlamydia pneumoniae*, a bacterium widespread among humans that often gets into the lungs and causes colds, but can also infect monocytes in the blood and settle in the walls of arteries. These studies have found a close relationship between infection caused by this bacterium and the risk of heart attack, so much so that in the 1990s cardiologists began to ask themselves whether heart disease might be caused by infection, just as today we know that stomach ulcers are not due to stress but to bacteria. But three major studies into the possibility of preventing heart attacks with antibiotics (with drugs that specifically fight bacteria) failed, whereas studies to prevent stomach ulcers with antibiotics were successful.

Today we know that chlamydia do not cause heart disease, that they are not responsible for cholesterol accumulating on artery walls, and that they are not the primary catalyst of atherosclerosis. They may, however, trigger a heart attack, probably because they infect monocytes and cause inflammation that increases the risk of clots.

Pollution and Other Triggers

Air pollution has also been shown, in over 150 studies in the past fifteen years, to be a contributor to cardiovascular accidents. It has been observed, for example, that people living less than 100 meters (328 feet) from a highway or less than 50 meters (164 feet) from a busy downtown street are twice as likely to die from cardiorespiratory disease than the rest of the population. As far as the heart itself is concerned, it has been suggested that pollution from fine particles such as those emitted by motor vehicles may have the capacity to trigger heart attacks and arrhythmias, damage artery walls, and increase blood clotting.

In one study we did in our laboratory at Mount Sinai Hospital in New York City, we found that no extreme pollution episodes are needed to cause such damage to the heart, but rather they may occur at pollution levels we accept as normal. And we have begun another study with people working at highway tolls, who are exposed to high levels of vehicle emissions on a daily basis, to assess the impact of air pollution on blood and arterial inflammation. We have not yet completed the puzzle. We are still fitting together the pieces that would give us a better understanding of the relationship between air pollution and cardiovascular health. But the picture that emerges is that the more pollution, the higher the risk. And just as we have reduced the levels we consider acceptable for cholesterol and high blood pressure, I believe we are headed for a future where, as we gain knowledge of the impact of air pollution on health, we will also lower the levels that are considered acceptable.

Another potential trigger for an inflammatory reaction in the blood and/or arterial wall (although we have less data on this than on pollution) is the sort of eating binge rich in animal fats and sugars we are especially prone to indulge in on holidays such as Thanksgiving or Christmas. Though an infrequent occurrence, it is not unheard of for someone with damaged coronary arteries to be struck down upon leaving a restaurant after a copious meal. And this probably happens because after the meal, the level of triglycerides in the blood skyrockets and causes an acute blood inflammation that promotes clotting. By contrast, the type of local inflammation that occurs when a person suffers a blow, sprain, or fracture has nothing to do with blood or arterial inflammation and has no appreciable bearing on the risk of a heart attack.

In Search of a Good Marker

Ultimately, the conclusion that emerges from all this data we have been gathering, all these pieces to the puzzle that are forming an increasingly coherent picture, is that inflammation is no less important than cholesterol or hypertension in the origin of cardiovascular disease. However, although it is recommended that everyone over twenty years of age have their cholesterol and blood pressure checked on a regular basis, it is not yet recommended that they test for blood inflammation. Why not?

In fact, there is a test to measure blood inflammation. What the test actually measures is the level of a substance called C-reactive protein (CRP). CRP is what we call an inflammation marker: the more pronounced the inflammation, the higher the level of this protein. It has been observed that CRP level helps define a person's risk of heart attack.

But as a marker, it is somewhat imprecise because high CRP does not always mean high cardiovascular risk. In some cases, it does indeed reflect an inflammation of the arteries or blood. But in other cases it may reflect a cold, a sports injury, or some other type of blood inflammation that triggers an elevated secretion of CRP but has no significance with regard to cardiovascular health.

With LDL cholesterol or blood pressure, things are much clearer: a high level always means high cardiovascular risk. Until we find a perfect marker, CRP testing remains restricted to people who have a history of coronary problems or cardiovascular risk factors associated with inflammation, such as diabetes or hypercholesterolemia. In these cases, high CRP is an additional warning signal to be extra careful. But the CRP test is not recommended for healthy people who have no reason to suspect that they are at risk of suffering a heart attack.

When to Resort to Drugs

If inflammation is such a major factor in cardiovascular accidents, it may seem a good idea to prescribe anti-inflammatory drugs to prevent embolism and stroke.

In fact, aspirin's great effectiveness in cardiovascular prevention appears to be due not only to the fact that it prevents blood clotting, as we have long known. I believe that what explains its effectiveness is that it also acts as an anti-inflammatory on the blood.

And I doubt that the great effectiveness of statins is due solely to their impact on LDL cholesterol; probably it is due in part to the fact that they reduce inflammation. This would explain why statins may be effective against certain neurodegenerative diseases (something that is still under study as we have yet to come to any conclusive findings) and why statins may be effective against inflammatory diseases such as arthritis.

We are discovering that the impact of inflammation on health goes far beyond cardiovascular disease; how far, we do not yet know, and this is an exciting field of current research.

Of course, all this does not justify taking anti-inflammatory drugs indiscriminately as a preventive measure. So-called coxibs, for example, which in their day were lauded as an advance on aspirin and which include some of the best-known anti-inflammatories, are harmful to cardiovascular health. If you want to fight inflammation as a means of preventing heart attack, the last thing I would prescribe is an anti-inflammatory from the coxib family.

Aspirin neutralizes two substances: cox–1, which promotes blood clotting, and cox–2, which inhibits clotting. But coxibs have no effect on cox–1 and neutralize only cox–2, which means they favor rather than inhibit coagulation, thereby increasing the risk of clots. Of course, the ideal anti-inflammatory to prevent cardiovascular disease would do exactly the opposite: inhibit only cox–1 and leave cox–2 alone, thereby reducing the risk of clots.

But until we come up with such a drug, the best the patient can do to reduce cardiovascular inflammation is to fight the four major causes of inflammation, namely obesity, tobacco, LDL cholesterol, and excess blood sugar. And to do so, three things suffice: watch your diet, exercise, and do not smoke.

Ultimately, after so many years studying cardiovascular disease, one realizes that there are myriad factors that may lead to heart attack: factors ranging from hypertension to high cholesterol to inflammation to diabetes; factors that produce extremely complex situations in your arteries, with hundreds of proteins involved in ultrafast biochemical reactions, taking place in fractions of a second. But all these problems, as diverse and complex as they are, lead to but one solution: healthy diet, physical exercise, and no smoking.

That's all: just these three basic tips. So simple it catches a lot of people unaware.

CHAPTER NINE

Vitamins and Minerals

WHY DOCTORS RECOMMEND EATING FRUIT

Now that we've seen the many ways in which obesity, tobacco, high cholesterol, hypertension, and inflammation cause natural disasters in our body, it may be comforting to recall that there is a whole series of small pleasures that are good for your heart. A bit of chocolate, a glass of wine, garlic soup, a handful of walnuts. . .Small pleasures rich in antioxidants that help limit the damage of chemical residues that the human body produces endlessly.

Danger: Free Radicals

The human body is actually a prodigious chemical machine. It feeds itself oxygen through the lungs and food through the digestive system. It processes everything in complex reactions to obtain the raw materials it needs to regenerate and the energy it needs to function, and like any chemical machine, it generates waste.

This waste includes free radicals, which are formed naturally by the human body's own metabolism. These molecules lack an electron, making them unstable, aggressive, and prone to thieving. In search of stability, they steal electrons from neighboring molecules, which in turn become free radicals themselves and thus hijack other molecules for their electrons. Thus arises a gang of free radicals stealing electrons from each other in what we call oxidation reactions. Free radicals are currently blamed for atherosclerosis, Alzheimer's, osteoporosis, most types of diabetes, some cancers, and the entire aging process—in short, the very causes of the vast majority of deaths.

Fortunately, the human body has what we might call a police force out there twenty-four hours a day hunting down free radicals. These cops are the antioxidants we get from a diet that contains foods such as chocolate, wine, garlic, and, above all, fruit and vegetables. Antioxidants are molecules that give an electron to the free radicals to rehabilitate them, without turning corrupt in the process since they themselves remain chemically stable even minus an electron.

In a healthy person, the antioxidant corps is capable of containing the action of free radicals. In some organ, a crime is always being committed, theft of an electron, an unarrested oxidation, but the body of a healthy person is not a lawless land. However, when free radicals grow faster than the antioxidant police's ability to contain them, the criminal element gains the upper hand and can cause enormous damage.

In terms of cardiovascular disease, free radicals oxidize LDL cholesterol, they injure artery walls, and they block the body's defenses against atherosclerosis. And the more extensive the damage—for example, the more oxidized LDL cholesterol there is in the blood—the greater the risk of heart attack. Especially vulnerable to such harm are smokers and perhaps people exposed to certain types of radiation or high levels of pollution because these are factors that produce free radicals.

The above factors notwithstanding, there are also people whose diet is simply too poor in antioxidants to control the free radicals the body produces naturally. In these cases, of course, the best thing they can do is try to get more antioxidants.

A Brief Guide to Antioxidants

Before you run off to grab a piece of fruit or raid the chocolates shelf at the supermarket, you should realize that there are different types of antioxidants: not all act alike and there are big differences from one food to another in terms of antioxidant power.

Among the several antioxidants most closely linked to cardiovascular prevention is vitamin E, which is abundant in vegetable oils such as olive or sunflower and nuts such as almonds and hazelnuts. It has been shown that people who have a diet rich in vitamin E also have a lower risk of heart attack, although we have yet to clarify whether vitamin E is the key or whether we are simply dealing with people who eat well in general. Probably both are true: vitamin E is heart-healthy and someone who has a diet rich in vitamin E tends to be someone who takes care of themselves. Intriguingly, contrary to the likely benefit of vitamin E contained in natural food, studies on vitamin E supplements have not shown the same benefit, and some have even found a tendency to harm.

By definition, a vitamin is a substance that the human body is unable to produce, so we must get it from food. Vitamin E is the most important of the fat-soluble antioxidants, which evidently are not found in fruits and vegetables but rather in some foods rich in fat.

As for the water-soluble antioxidants, which are abundant in fruits and vegetables, the most important is vitamin C. Studies into whether vitamin C prevents cardiovascular disease have provided no conclusive findings. It may aid prevention, but we do not have the proof to make a definitive claim. Nor is it clear whether it does anything to prevent or treat colds, despite the volume of vitamin C sold each winter in pharmacies. What is clear is that vitamin C is a great antioxidant and that when you don't have enough of it, health problems appear.

The best sources of vitamin C are fruits and vegetables. Among fruits: strawberries, kiwifruit, and oranges. Vegetables, especially those of the cruciferous family, such as broccoli, cabbage, and cauliflower, are also high in vitamin C. But because it is vulnerable to heat, anyone who wants to conserve not just vitamins but most of the nutrients in their vegetables may want to steam rather than boil.

A third type of important antioxidant, after vitamins E and C, are carotenoids, which are abundant in red and orange vegetables such as carrots and tomatoes. The name *carotenoid* actually shares its etymological root with carrot (also *carotte* in French, for instance), and among the substances in the carotenoid group we find beta-carotene, which is what gives carrots their orange color, besides being a powerful antioxidant.

More powerful still appears to be lycopene, which gives tomatoes their red color and which is not destroyed by cooking and is especially abundant in fried tomatoes and ketchup.

A Picasso on Every Plate

Orange beta-carotene, red lycopene. . .When one stops to think about it, the color of fruits and vegetables may just be more important than would seem at first glance.

As a general rule, the more colorful the vegetable, the richer it will be in antioxidants. This rule is not infallible; there are exceptions. But color is so important that the American Heart Association, after reviewing all we know today about antioxidants, explicitly recommends "habitually consuming a variety of fruits and vegetables, especially those that are dark green, deep orange, or yellow" (Fig. 8).

As for fruit, although the appeal may be in the skin color, what matters most is the color of the flesh, the part you eat. Watermelon, for example, contains more lycopene than melon. Peaches and oranges are high in antioxidants. Dark green broccoli has more than its pallid cousin cauliflower. Which is not to say that white-fleshed fruits such as apples or pears are less nutritious. On the contrary, they are very healthy and have many other virtues, such as large amounts of fiber, but they are relatively low in antioxidants.

Say you are making a salad. Take a pale green iceberg lettuce and dress with oil and vinegar: highly recommended. But, in addition to all the benefits of the fiber and minerals in lettuce, if you want to get the rewards of antioxidants, the best thing you can do is to make your plate look like a Picasso or a Kandinsky. Perhaps start with a background of lettuce, then add brushstrokes of red, orange, green, yellow, with touches of bell pepper (which has an extraordinary amount of antioxidants), tomato, carrot, beet. . . . Ultimately, your best bet is to be creative and treat your plate as if it were a work of art.

20 Grams of Fiber a Day

In fact, the benefits of fruits and vegetables go well beyond antioxidants. They also provide folic acid, which is essential during pregnancy and child development. They provide a wide variety of minerals and vitamins. They provide a long list of healthy substances with complicated names: flavonoids, polyphenols, glucosinolate, organosulfates, terpenes. . . . And they contain a good amount of fiber, an important complex carbohydrate.

Apples, for example, are loaded with pectin, a fiber that blocks sugar and cholesterol in food from passing into the blood, and thus helps fight diabetes and high cholesterol. In addition, fiber gives you a feeling of being full, which is good for people who are overweight or obese.

Broadly speaking, there are two types of fibers. Soluble fibers such as pectin, which dissolve in water and help control blood sugar and blood cholesterol. And non-soluble fibers, which ease food through the digestive system and help prevent constipation. Both come from plant foods, not just fruits and vegetables but also pulses, such as chickpeas or lentils, and whole grains. And both are very effective allies in the battle against cardiovascular disorders.

However, the amount of fiber most people in Western countries eat remains well below the recommended 20 grams a day—a rough target easily reached with a bowl of whole grain cereal for breakfast (5 grams), a plate of vegetables with a potato at lunchtime (another 5 grams), an apple for dessert (5 grams), and with dinner, a salad (just over 5 grams). For those who want more, a dish of lentils or chickpeas would provide about another 20 grams of fiber, and a 50-gram snack of nuts is worth 4 grams of insurance.

Chocolate, Reputation Restored

Even chocolate can be a good source of fiber. Which is not to say you should try to get your daily 20 grams munching on chocolate bars. But 10 grams of dark chocolate provides 2 grams of fiber as healthy as that in fruit, potatoes, or whole grains. Chocolate comes from a plant, which is why it is a healthy food. Its basic ingredient is cocoa beans, a complex, highly sophisticated fruit with a number of extraordinary properties.

By adding sugar and cutting it with milk and cocoa butter, Western culture has turned chocolate into little more than candy. But studies into the nutritive properties of cocoa and its impact on health are restoring its reputation. It has even been calculated that eating dark chocolate daily may reduce the risk of heart attack. And some studies suggest that flavonoids in chocolate, just as in tea or fruit, may help lower blood pressure.

But to get these benefits, and this is a key point, the chocolate must be high in cocoa. The lower the cocoa content and the higher the sugar, the less the health benefits, no matter how dark the chocolate. And if instead of being dark, it's white or milk chocolate, it will provide no appreciable benefit to your health (although it will do no harm either, as long as it is eaten in moderation).

A second key point is that chocolate, even when it contains little sugar, is a calorie bomb. So if you eat a lot of chocolate, you should cut down on the calories you get elsewhere.

Other foods, which, like chocolate, are known to be heart-healthy and are now recommended, often in moderation, include: wine (which may reduce the risk of heart attack, so long as you drink no more than one to two glasses a day); garlic (which contains a variety of antioxidants); nuts (which may reduce risk thanks not only to antioxidants but also to their healthy fats); and fish (which also contains healthy fats).

Recommendation Number One

Eating well is so important to health that when I was president of the American Heart Association, a panel of nineteen experts reviewed all the available scientific evidence on the relationship between diet and cardiovascular disease and drew up a list of recommendations that remain valid today.

Recommendation number one is: "Eat a variety of fruits and vegetables at least five times each day." A diet rich in vegetables, the panel found, reduces the risk of heart disease, stroke, hypertension, and obesity. Five servings may seem like a lot, but we are not talking about especially large servings. Each piece of fruit, for example, is considered one serving. A salad or vegetables to go with a main dish is considered another serving. A whole plate of salad would be two servings. So five servings a day is not impossible (Fig. 8).

But in the Western world we are not reaching that target. Not only are we not getting those five servings but we are actually moving in the opposite direction. Even in a Mediterranean county like Spain, 36 percent of the population, more than 1 in 3 people, does not eat fresh fruit every day. And the trend is toward eating less and less. According to a survey done in Catalonia, average fruit consumption per person has declined by 10 percent in ten years, vegetable consumption has fallen by 8 percent; fish, by 14 percent. In contrast, consumption of commercial juices containing large amounts of sugar has risen by 93 percent and baked goods by 20 percent.

These figures represent trends for the whole population and do not apply to every individual. There are millions of people in Spain who eat right. But when you look at what is happening with the population as a whole, you see that the diet is getting less Mediterranean and less healthy. And we have the great paradox of a society that eats too much but does not get enough vitamins.

Vitamin Supplements? No Thanks

If the trend is so negative, it would seem advisable to take vitamin supplements to compensate for the lack of antioxidants in our diet. But I do not believe supplements are a good idea.

The panel of experts that examined the pros and cons of different diets for the American Heart Association concluded that vitamin supplements with antioxidants have not been shown to be effective at all for cardiovascular prevention; the only thing that has proven effective is a diet rich in vegetables.

On the other hand, some of these supplements have been shown to have dangerous side effects, including higher risk of lung cancer in smokers who took the antioxidant beta-carotene.

So, given the absence of proof of effectiveness of vitamin supplements and the absence of proof that they are safe, it is wiser not to recommend them.

The only exception is folic acid, a vitamin that is plentiful in vegetables with lots of color such as spinach, pumpkins, green beans, and red peppers. Such supplements are recommended for all women who are planning to have a baby because a folic acid deficiency entails a risk of malformations in the development of the fetus in the early weeks of pregnancy, even before the woman knows she is pregnant. Folic acid is no longer recommended for people with cardiovascular disease and high levels of homocysteine, since it does not lower risk for cardiovascular disease.

But there are other exceptions. When a healthy person asks me, as often happens (with, for example, a man with no health problems who is unhappy about the physical decline that comes with aging), if I would advise them to take vitamin supplements to feel stronger, I always say that in their place I would not. "But won't they help me feel better?" they may insist. They may help, but it has not been proven that they will. In fact, in this situation supplements have not been shown either to work or not to work. So they may actually work. But we do not have the complete picture of antioxidants, and since some of the evidence shows that antioxidant supplements may even be dangerous, I tell them that in their place I would not take them.

What I would do is make sure I get enough antioxidants by eating plenty of fruits and vegetables.

Mineral Supplements? In Some Cases, Yes

Mineral supplements are a different matter. Like vitamins, minerals are nutrients the human body needs but is unable to manufacture, so we must get them from the food we eat. And when a person's diet does not supply enough minerals, it has been shown that certain supplements prevent serious health problems.

In the case of cardiovascular diseases, a lack of potassium and magnesium, found mainly in fruits and vegetables and fish, is associated with higher risk of cardiac arrhythmias. An iron deficiency, for example anemia, limits the amount of oxygen reaching the heart cells and can make angina or heart attack, should they occur, worse. In addition, low iron causes blood to flow faster, which puts a strain on the heart and can also aggravate heart disease. All these cases justify mineral supplements. But before you resort to supplements, an adequate diet is always preferable as a means of getting all the vitamins and minerals your body needs.

Is There Really an Ideal Diet?

An adequate diet must be varied and balanced, which means it can include just about any food (Fig. 8). Despite all the bad press beef has been getting for the saturated fats it contains, an ideal diet can include the occasional steak, which is also an excellent source of iron to prevent anemia and of vitamin E. It may include two eggs a week, providing magnesium, potassium, folic acid, and all the vitamins, minerals, proteins, and fats an embryo needs to develop. It may even include, now and then, a hotdog, bacon and eggs, or a croissant.

In other words there is no one ideal diet. Rather, there are many possible ideal diets with plenty of menus to choose from. They tend to follow certain rules, of course. They are often rich in complex carbohydrates, such as rice, lentils, bread, or potatoes, and they are low in sugars. Most of them favor healthy fats, such as those found in fish and olive oil, over the unhealthy fats, such as those in red meat and factory baked goods. And they are often high in fruits and vegetables. But within these rules, we have a vast range of choice so that anyone can find combinations of foods that are both healthy and suit their tastes. Overall, the key of a good diet can be simplified, "variety in quality and decrease in quantity."

figure 8

FOOD PYRAMID

Nutrition specialists illustrate the composition of an optimal diet with a six-level pyramid. Each level corresponds with a food group. The wider the level, the more frequently you should consume from that particular food group.

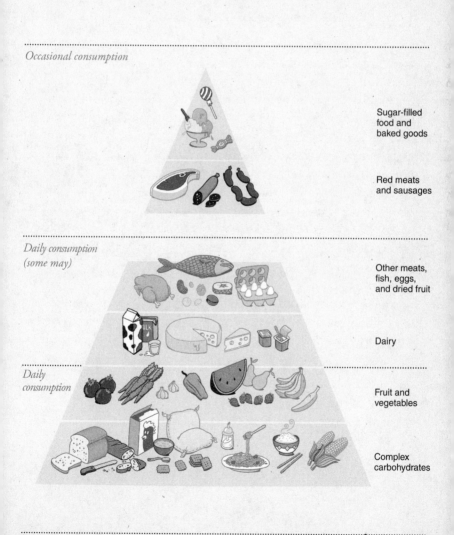

Occasional consumption

Sugar-filled food and baked goods

Red meats and sausages

Daily consumption (some may)

Other meats, fish, eggs, and dried fruit

Dairy

Daily consumption

Fruit and vegetables

Complex carbohydrates

CHAPTER TEN

Fat

DANGEROUS PLEASURES

Despite their bad reputation, fats have one major virtue: they are delicious. A dash of olive oil and a handful of nuts can turn an insipid salad into an excellent main dish. A chicken leg is more tender and tasty than a breast, which has less fat. To many palates, a butter croissant is tastier than a slice of bread. We might as well admit it—humans are designed to like fat. And one may think that nature is wise: thanks in large part to fat, an act as vital as eating food is a pleasure. A taste for fat is one of the gifts that nature has given us to protect us from malnutrition.

But today we have more food than we need within easy reach. Go into any supermarket and you enter a cornucopia of products in colorful packaging crying out: eat me! And just as the hunter-gatherers of the rain forests filled their baskets with fruits of appealing colors, the twenty-first-century consumer is prone to fill their shopping cart with whatever happens to catch their eye.

That's all fine and good. It is wonderful to be able to eat what you like and wonderful that hardly anyone now dies of hunger in the West. But the pendulum has swung the other way. We no longer die from a lack of food; we die because we have too much.

The problem is that the human body needs just the right amount of each food to function in that state of equilibrium we call health. If you do not eat, you get sick; if you eat too much, you get sick, too. Cells manufacture cholesterol because they need it likewise, you can not live with too much cholesterol. It's the same with sugar, fat, salt, even water. Health is a state of equilibrium, and when you give free rein to your instincts and eat everything you can get your hands on, you upset that balance and that is where disease starts.

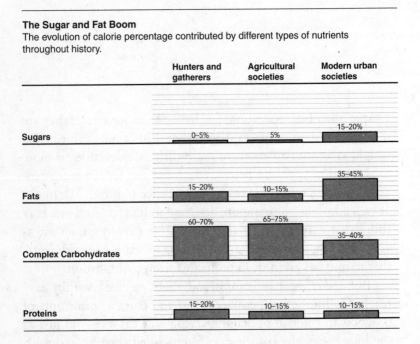

The Sugar and Fat Boom
The evolution of calorie percentage contributed by different types of nutrients throughout history.

	Hunters and gatherers	Agricultural societies	Modern urban societies
Sugars	0–5%	5%	15–20%
Fats	15–20%	10–15%	35–45%
Complex Carbohydrates	60–70%	65–75%	35–40%
Proteins	15–20%	10–15%	10–15%

Our instincts are not going to save us from imbalance or protect our health because following our instincts leads to excess. And this excess is not only with regard to eating; nor is it solely a matter of health. We are also prone to excess when it comes to money, power, the desire to possess, the desire to dominate. Our civilization as a whole tends toward imbalance, toward illness, toward self-destruction. And the only cure we have, the only resources we have to defend ourselves, are education and rationality. They are our only two medicines.

So, returning to fats, in order to make rational decisions that help us protect our health, it may be useful to know that they fall into five major groups and that each group acts in a different way in the human body. To avoid using too many technical terms, we will define each by a representative foodstuff: olive oil (monounsaturated fat); sunflower oil (polyunsaturated omega 6); fish (polyunsaturated omega 3); beef (saturated); and factory baked goods (trans fats). Although they all fit into a balanced diet, the first three (unsaturated) are considered healthy fats, whereas the last two (saturated and trans) are unhealthy and should be consumed only in moderation.

Monounsaturated: Olive Oil

In fact, for the human machine to function properly, fats are essential. We need them to build cell membranes, to manufacture hormones, for our immune system, for reproduction, even to think. The latter is especially true of babies and children, who need fats for proper brain development. But in adults, too, fats are essential to communication between neurons. They are so important that the American Heart Association recommends up to 30 percent of the calories you eat can come from fat.

Of that 25–30 percent it is recommended that approximately half be monounsaturated fats, which predominate in olive oil, making it ideal for salad dressing and cooking. Its main virtue is that relative to saturated fat in the general American diet, it lowers LDL cholesterol (lousy) and slightly raises HDL (healthy). Olive oil also provides vitamin E and other antioxidants.

And it is one of the basic ingredients in the Mediterranean diet, one of the healthiest diets in the world, although we do not know to what extent olive oil is responsible for its being so healthy. It's like a winning football team—who can say what share of the merit for victory goes to each player? The same is true of the Mediterranean diet: it might win the health game, but we cannot separate the benefits of olive oil from those of cereals, vegetables, or a glass of wine. The important thing, rather than each separate ingredient, is the whole.

Among the foods that provide significant amounts of monounsaturated fats are nuts such as hazelnuts, almonds, or macadamia nuts; some fish such as cod, mackerel, and herring; some poultry, such as chicken and duck; and avocados. These are all recommended foods for a healthy diet, but like all fatty foods, they have the disadvantage of being high in calories, which may cause some confusion for people trying to make the correct dietary choices.

I remember a patient who told me: "Doctor, first you tell me to eat less fat, and then you say eat more olive oil. But if the oil is a fat, what should I do?"

Indeed, every gram of fat contains nine calories, while a gram of protein or carbohydrates contains four. So, if you want to control cholesterol, it is best to include foods rich in monounsaturated fats in your diet. But if you want to control your weight, you should consume them in moderation.

So I told him: "You should do both. You should cut down on fat because you are overweight and your diet is too high in fats, which have lots of calories. That is the most important thing. But besides that it would do you good to replace part of the saturated fats you eat, such as in meat and sausage, with unsaturated fats" (Fig. 8).

Polyunsaturated Omega–6: Sunflower Oil

While olive oil is rich in monounsaturated fats, other vegetable oils are richer in polyunsaturated fats called omega–6. Examples are sunflower oil, corn oil, safflower oil, which reduces total blood cholesterol even more than olive oil does, but has the disadvantage of reducing both LDL (bad) and HDL (good). Another major drawback is that this type of fat is unsuitable for cooking, especially for frying because heat degrades it and turns it into unhealthy fat. Apart from sunflower oil, other vegetable oils such as corn or soybean are rich in omega–6 fats, as are walnuts, pine nuts, and sunflower seeds.

The few rigorous studies that have been done on the benefits of this type of fat suggest—but do not prove—that they are good for cardiovascular accident prevention, especially in people with diabetes. This may be due to omega–6 fats enhancing the effectiveness of insulin in regulating blood sugar, in addition to their direct impact on cholesterol, but we need more research in order to confirm this.

The truth is that, today, we do not know how much omega–6 fat an ideal diet should include. We know that the human body cannot manufacture such facts, so we have to get at least a small amount from the food we eat. But we do not know what happens when they are ingested in large amounts: whether a diet rich in omega–6 would lessen the effects of diabetes or, conversely, have an adverse impact in the long term.

There are so many questions and so little data that for now the American Heart Association recommends a diet in which no more than 10 percent of calories come from this type of fat. For cooking, the AHA recommends avoiding oils rich in omega–6, like sunflower, and using olive oil instead.

Polyunsaturated Omega–3: Oily Fish

On the other hand, we have lots of studies and lots of evidence that the fats characteristic of oily fish, omega–3s, are a real blessing for your health, especially cardiovascular health.

These fats, about which we knew next to nothing twenty years ago, have turned out to be a sort of miracle food. We cannot say whether they are better or worse than those in olive oil, only that they are complementary. So, what we can say is that both are essential in a balanced diet.

We did not realize the immense benefits of a diet rich in omega–3 until the 1980s, when it was discovered that people who eat fish regularly as the Eskimos do are significantly less likely to die from heart disease than people who rarely eat fish.

Since then, many studies have confirmed the benefits of omega–3 fats; others have not. The major benefits have been shown among people who already suffer heart disease. Indeed, doctors need to give such people dietary advice tailored to their particular needs, rather than just the same old advice we give a healthy person: in people with cardiovascular problems we have seen that weekly consumption of about a half pound of fish significantly reduces the risk of sudden death. It has also been shown that, in addition to protecting against cardiovascular disease, omega–3s help fight certain autoimmune and inflammatory diseases.

We do not know exactly how they work. It has been shown that they lower triglycerides and improve the lipid profile of the blood, which is good but does not explain all of their salutary effects. We know they reduce clotting in the blood, and hence the risk of stroke and heart attack—bearing in mind that the direct cause of either one is a clot. And they reduce the risk of arrhythmia, which explains why they prevent sudden death in heart patients.

But although we do not understand why, omega–3s are so beneficial that today the American Heart Association recommends that everyone eat fish at least twice a week. For cardiovascular patients the recommendation is to eat fish more often or take omega–3 supplements in doses of up to 850 milligrams daily. The fish richest in omega–3, and thus the healthiest, are oily fish such as salmon, tuna, anchovies, sardines, or herring.

Significant amounts of omega–3 are also found in plants such as nuts, soybean, and rapeseed. All these can be considered heart-healthy foods.

On the contrary, there is no evidence that foods fortified with omega–3 now sold in supermarkets, such as milk or eggs, have any beneficial effects at all in the long run. The fact that we lack the evidence does not mean that they are not beneficial; it just means we do not know because we need more data.

So when someone asks me: "Doctor, should I buy milk with omega–3?" I say that I do not think it does any harm.

But if you're worried about getting enough omega–3, the best thing you can do is eat fish, oily fish if possible, at least twice a week. The fish, I can assure you, will help preserve your health; as for the milk, I cannot say.

Saturated: Red Meat

Now that we have dealt with the three types of healthy fats—olive oil and fish (unquestionably good) and sunflower oil (less certain)—it is time to enter the dangerous terrain of saturated fats, associated with red meat and other animal products. With the monounsaturates in olive oil and omega–3 in fish, the basic recommendation is to consume more. Here the basic recommendation is to consume less. And there are good reasons for this: too much saturated fat is the number one cause of the high levels of LDL cholesterol (bad) so common in Western countries.

Many studies have shown that the higher the consumption of saturated fats in a society, the greater the risk of heart attack. Moreover, too much red meat and saturated fats increases the risk of colorectal cancer by about 30 percent and, in women, the risk of breast cancer by about 15 percent. It is also likely to increase the risk of esophageal and gastric cancers, although the data we have here is less conclusive.

The case against saturated fats is so strong that the American Heart Association recommends a diet in which no more than 10 percent of calorie intake comes from this class of fats. That would mean a substantial reduction compared with current levels of consumption. People diagnosed with a cardiovascular condition are advised to be even stricter and to lower their relative intake of saturated fats to 7 percent.

Achieving these levels is not always easy in countries where eating red meat, sausages, and dairy products such as cheese, butter, and cream is ingrained in the culinary culture. When you have been eating meat daily all your life, changing your habits can be tough.

I remember the case of a patient who told me: "You know, doctor? I did as you told me, and I don't eat nearly as much fat."

"Congratulations," I said. "And what do you eat now?"

"Well, I still eat more or less the same things, but now when I have a steak, I am careful to cut off all the fat."

The man was right to reduce the amount of saturated fat he ate. It's a good idea to trim the large chunks of fat from meat. But although he did not know it, he was still eating too much saturated fat. The problem is that you cannot see about half the fats in meat. They are in the cell membranes and spaces between cells, so, though they make meat more tender and tasty, you end up eating a lot more fat than you may actually realize. So, when you trim off the visible fat before digging in, you only reduce the amount of fat by half.

There are also invisible fats in eggs, milk, baked ham, and, generally speaking, in nearly all animal products. When you have a glass of milk or coffee with milk, you'd hardly know by the appearance or taste how much fat you are ingesting. So, if you cannot always tell by looking, what rule of thumb can our patient follow to further reduce his intake of saturated fats?

"What you could do is eat less animal products, with the exception of fish," I advised him. "Instead of doing as you have always done, having meat as your main dish every day, why not try starting with salad and then have a plate of pasta, rice, or beans? And what you can also do, if you are going to eat meat and dairy products, is pick foods that are already low in fats, such as lean meats or low-fat or no-fat milk, yogurt, or cheese (Fig. 8). Anyway," I told him, "there is a type of fat that is even worse than saturated that we eat too much of."

Examples of Foods Rich in Fat
The numbers indicate the content, in grams, of the different
nutrients for every 100 grams of food.

	Carbohydrates	Fats	Proteins
Fatty cheese (Roquefort)	0	31	21
Parmesan cheese	0	26	36
Cream	3.5	32	2.5
Sausages	1	27	13
Nuts and dried fruits	11	62	12
Olives	2	14	1.5
Liver pâté	1	29	13
Butter	0	80	0

Trans Fats: Factory Baked Goods

These fats, the undisputed champions of unhealthiness, are
called trans fat acids. You may find them on food labeling under
the name of hydrogenated vegetable fats, which is correct but
misleading because it may lead some consumers to relate vegetable fats with good health, when in fact hydrogenated fats are
harmful.

Unlike saturated fats, of which the human body needs a
small amount, trans fats have no virtues at all in terms of health.
On the contrary, they are bad for you in a number of ways: they
raise bad cholesterol, they lower good cholesterol, they increase
triglycerides, which can interfere with insulin and so increase
the risk of diabetes, and they probably inhibit the capacity of
blood vessels to dilate.

The biggest study into the relationship between diet and cardiovascular risk, involving over eighty thousand women over a
period of fourteen years, revealed that trans fats are even worse
for your health than saturated fats. For every 2 percent increase
in calorie intake from trans fats in your diet—just 2 percent—
the risk of cardiovascular accident increases by 25 percent. If

they are so bad for your health, one may wonder what they are doing in the food we eat.

Trans fats are most prevalent in factory baked goods (cakes, cookies, pies, and muffins), in the fried food served by fast-food chains and many restaurants, in pre-prepared fried food, and in some margarines. And the reason they are in all these products has nothing to do with nutrition but everything to do with profit. First because trans fats are cheap and reusable. But above all because trans fats make food more appetizing. When baked goods are made with olive oil, which is liquid at room temperature, they turn oily. But when they are made with trans fats, you don't get dirty fingers. Since trans fats remain solid at room temperature, they hide in food, and it is difficult for consumers to know how much of the stuff there is in their cookies, cakes, frozen, fried, or precooked foods.

The United States has been a pioneer in protecting by law the right of consumers to know how much trans fats food contains. But in most countries, and this is something that still should be remedied, there is no comparable legislation and the food industry usually conceals trans fats under the name of vegetable fats, without telling you what percentage of these vegetable fats are artificially modified.

All this does not mean we must banish cookies and precooked food from our diet. All foods fit into a balanced diet and the American Heart Association accepts a diet in which trans fats account for a small amount of calorie intake, but no more than 2 percent. Two percent is not a lot. So the best thing you can do is follow the example of the Cookie Monster and switch to fruit; you can have a cookie once in a while but not every day as before.

Which Cooking Oil?

Now that you understand the five major types of fat, things get a little more complicated (don't panic, just a little) when it comes to cooking.

The problem is that heat triggers chemical reactions that alter fats. You do not need to be a chemist to see this. Hardly anyone would dress a salad with oil that had been used for frying; we are all aware of the difference between raw oil and oil from the skillet.

But heat does not affect all oils in the same way. Olive oil, which contains mostly monounsaturates, retains much of its nutritional qualities when used for frying. Polyunsaturates such as sunflower, by contrast, oxidize and quickly become unhealthy fats. The same happens if you fry with margarine, which is rich in polyunsaturated fats that become harmful when heated.

So, as a rule it is better to fry with olive oil than margarine or sunflower oil. And whatever you use, it is not a good idea to refry oil many times over. If it has been used to fry meat, the oil will be loaded with saturated fats; if it has been used for frying potatoes, heat causes chemical reactions that degrade oil.

A healthier alternative to frying is to grill, boil, roast, or bake. Grilling liquefies the fat in meat or fish, which means less fat and fewer calories, and thus is recommended for overweight people. Boiled food is especially low in fat and thus easy to digest, and so doctors recommend it for people with digestive disorders. The disadvantage is that because the temperature is so high, boiling destroys some of the vitamins in vegetables. Another option is to steam, which does not destroy so many vitamins.

In short, there are many possible ways to cook your food, each with its pros and cons. But if you do not have health problems, I would say that you should enjoy—within reason, especially in the case of fried food—your very human appreciation of the delicious taste of fats.

CHAPTER ELEVEN

Proteins

NATURAL BORN CARNIVORES

It's part of getting old: there comes a time in everyone's life when they start to feel vulnerable. Around the time you hit fifty or so you realize you no longer have as much energy as before. You don't look so good in the mirror, with gray hairs and wrinkles. You start getting aches and pains. You are no longer that surfer riding the crest of the wave— And one of the most common reactions, as I have seen from my patients, is to become obsessed with your health. Around seventy-five, when they realize that time is running out, people often tend to ask themselves transcendental questions and more than ever seek answers in religion. But among fifty-year-olds, an age at which people are more worried about decline than death, I have come across patients who ask me how they can keep their vitality and youthful appearance. I remember a man who was willing to try anything to keep feeling young:

"Doctor," he asked, "do you think I should stop eating meat, you know, go vegetarian?"

It is the dream of eternal youth twenty-first-century version. In ancient times people made a deal with the devil—now they talk to their doctor.

Essential Amino Acids

Stop eating meat? Why not? Vegetarians rarely have the sort of cholesterol or weight problems that cause so many premature deaths in the West.

But before turning vegetarian you should know that meat is a major source of protein in our diet and that proteins are the building blocks of which the human body is made. Your bones, your muscles, your eyes, your skin—your entire body is built of proteins. And because the human body is always under construction, as millions of cells die every day and must be replaced, we also need to refuel on proteins every day.

Moreover, we use proteins to transport from one organ to another substances like the hemoglobin in your blood that carries oxygen all around your body. We use them in the form of hormones as a means of communication between organs, such as when the brain signals the ovaries to ovulate. Our immune system uses proteins to defend us from external threats. And they even provide a backup energy source should we ever run out of reserves of fat and carbohydrates (which is why starving people's bones and muscles waste away: they burn the protein in them).

So perhaps we can live without meat, but we cannot live without proteins. Each of the proteins in the human body is actually a highly complex three-dimensional construct, made up of components called amino acids. There are 22 different amino acids that our cells need to produce the thousands of proteins in our body. Just as all the words in a language can be formed out of the letters in its alphabet, we can form all our proteins with 22 amino acids. And the most important thing to know before becoming a vegetarian is that your body can synthesize 14 of those 22 amino acids, but you have to get the other 8 from the food you eat.

Those eight are called essential amino acids: trying to make your body function without one of these essential amino acids would be like trying to spell Mississippi without the letter *s*, or mother, macaroni, or moose without an *m*. Similarly, the lack of an essential amino acid is a sure ticket to disorders. The eight essential amino acids are abundant in animal products such as meat, fish, eggs, and milk. Of plant-based foods, though many do provide some proteins, and thus amino acids, only one, soybeans, contains all eight essentials.

Thus, unless you eat the right balance of vegetables to ensure an adequate supply of the eight essentials, a strict vegetarian diet, without eggs or milk, can lead to an insufficiency of amino acids (Fig. 8).

Protein Overdose

Still, it does not take vast amounts of protein to meet the needs of the human body. For a healthy adult, less than 1 gram of protein per kilogram (2.2 pounds) of body weight a day is enough. In other words, a person weighing 70 kilograms (154 pounds) needs no more than 70 grams (2.5 ounces) of protein daily. And of those 70 grams, a 50–50 balance between animal products and vegetables will cover all your daily needs for amino acids.

So if for lunch you have a 150 grams (5.3 ounce) steak, containing more than 100 grams of water and about 30 grams of protein, you will get almost enough animal protein to meet your needs for the entire day. If you have coffee with milk (5 grams of protein) with breakfast, low fat cottage cheese or yogurt or nuts as a snack or appetizer (another 10 grams), a plate of peas or pasta for lunch (another 10 to 15 grams), and chicken or fish (10 grams) for dinner, by the end of the day you'll have easily ingested more protein than you need.

In rare cases, too many proteins can overload your kidneys and impair their ability to remove excess urea from your blood. Too many proteins also favor calcium loss in your bones and increase the risk of osteoporosis. Nor is it uncommon for people with high protein diets to suffer gout due to excess uric acid in the blood, which can be very uncomfortable.

But the main problem associated with excess proteins is rarely the proteins themselves. The main problem is the saturated fats that you are getting along with the proteins in animal products. If you eat 300 grams (10.5 ounces) of meat a day, which is what the average European eats, you may also be getting 50 grams of fat in the deal. If you restrict your diet to chicken breasts and other lean meats, you will get less than 50 grams of fat. But if you like hamburgers and sausages, as many people do, you'll easily top that amount. Many types of sausages and cold cuts contain twice as much fat as protein.

These fats, in addition to the eggs, cheese, and other animal products many people eat in a day, raise the level of LDL cholesterol (bad) in your blood and increase the risk of cardiovascular disease, neurodegenerative diseases, and some cancers.

In the end one might come to the conclusion that we are not well adapted to a high-protein diet. Carnivores, lions or crocodiles, for instance, can eat as much meat as they like without ever getting a cholesterol problem. They are so well adapted to eating meat that research into new drugs against atherosclerosis is examining how cats and reptiles process fat. By contrast, herbivores cannot survive on a diet high in saturated fats. From this standpoint, we are closer to the herbivores than the carnivores. But we are not well adapted to a diet low in protein.

We became humans because we ate meat, as the study of human evolution shows. The first humans appeared 2.5 million years ago after hominids added meat to their diet. Until then, the Australopithecus vegetarian diet was a brake on the brain development of offspring during pregnancy, and our ancestors' brain never reached a size larger than that of a chimpanzee's. But from the moment hominids began to eat meat, with its high nutritional value, their brain began to grow in the prenatal stage to the point where, 2.5 million years later, we are born with a formidable brain, pre-programmed for language, music, and science, with a capacity that not even the most powerful super-computer in the world can match.

So here's the great paradox: that a diet rich in animal proteins was key to our birth as a species, while an excess of these same proteins often leads to our death as individuals. And perhaps what we should be asking ourselves is where to get the proteins we need to live, especially those eight essential amino acids, without paying the price in the form of a heart attack.

Meat or Fish?

Every time you go to the supermarket to shop for high-protein food, you are faced with the choice between the meat or the fish department. Both offer all eight essential amino acids, but they contain different types of fat in different proportions. The meat department has sources of lower and higher saturated fats: white meat of chicken, veal, and well-trimmed pork; lean cuts of beef that are lower in saturated fats; marbled beef, ribs, lamb chops that are higher.

By contrast, habitual consumption of fish has the opposite effect: not only does it not increase but it actually reduces the risk of cardiovascular accidents, as was discovered in studies of Inuit populations with extremely limited diets. We once believed that in the Arctic, where fruits and vegetables do not grow as they do in our climates, and the only food found in abundance is fish, especially the oily varieties, people would have huge rates of cardiovascular disease. But in the late 1970s we found to our surprise that heart attacks are rare among Inuit who base their diet on fish. Later, we discovered that this is probably due to the omega-3 fats in fish, which, as it turns out, have beneficial effects on your heart and arteries. So, as a rule, meats contain a type of fat that is harmful in abundance, whereas fish contain a type of fat that is healthy in abundance.

The Fish Conundrum: White or Oily?

Let's take a look, then, at the fish department. Here we find a variety of fish and shellfish that have different pros and cons with regard to our health. Fish can be divided into whitefish (such as monkfish, sole, hake, and cod) and oily fish (such as tuna, sardines, and salmon). They all have a lot of what we call high biological value protein, which is a way of saying they contain all eight essential amino acids. And they all provide omega–3 fats.

The big difference between white and oily fish is in the amount of fat they contain. For example, 100 grams (3.5 ounces) of tuna contain about 15 grams of fat; 100 grams of sole or cod contain barely 1 gram. So, to achieve maximum cardiovascular benefit, oily is better than white because it provides more omega–3. But if your primary concern is overweight or obesity, whitefish may be better since it contains less fat.

However, fish fats have one drawback: this is where toxic substances such as mercury or organochlorine compounds accumulate. Hence, the more fish you eat, the more toxic chemicals you are exposed to. We do not know at what point the risks associated with the toxins outweigh the benefits of the fish. But we do know that when a big fish eats a small fish, the toxins in the prey end up in the predator's fat. So, the bigger the fish, generally speaking, the higher the concentration of toxins. With this in mind, it is wise to limit your consumption of large marine predators such as tuna or swordfish and eat more of the smaller oily fish such as mackerel or sardines. It is also wise for pregnant and nursing women to avoid large oily fish because the toxins they may contain are potentially damaging to a child's developing nervous system. Similarly, you should not introduce this sort of fish into your child's diet.

But aside from the above exceptions, eating oily fish at least twice a week is recommended for all people because, at that rate, the benefits far outweigh the potential risks.

As for shellfish, it contains very little fat, so it does not offer the same cardiovascular benefits as oily fish. And certain shell-fish, shrimp, and squid are high in cholesterol. One hundred grams of squid, for example, contains 170 milligrams of cholesterol, more than half the recommended daily maximum of 300 milligrams for a healthy person. But, other than shrimp and squid, which should be eaten in moderation, shellfish has the same advantage as whitefish: high-quality protein without raising the level of cholesterol in your blood.

Examples of Food Rich in Proteins
The numbers indicate the content, in grams, of the different nutrients for every 100 grams of food.

	Carbohydrates	Fats	Protein
Veal (steak)	0	5	21
Chicken (skinless breast)	0	1.5	21
Pork (loin)	0	4	22
Lamb	0	14	28
Whitefish (hake)	0	1	17
Shellfish (shrimp)	0	15	21
Shellfish (prawn)	0	1.5	19
Yogurt	4.5	4	4
Milk (low fat)	4.5	1.5	3.5
Eggs	0.5	11	13
Soy (weighed as dry bean)	6	18	34

The Meat Conundrum: Red or White?

After picking our fish, we now move on to the meat section. Here we have a choice: red meat (veal, beef, lamb); white meat (poultry—chicken, turkey), or pork. All three, within limits, have their place in a balanced diet (Fig. 8).

Red meat has the great virtue of containing lots of iron. Indeed what makes beef and lamb red is an iron-rich protein called myoglobin. It is also a type of iron that the body absorbs easily, unlike that in spinach (despite Popeye's claims for the stuff) and other vegetables, most of which is lost. So, the occasional steak or beef stew, say once a week, is recommended for people prone to anemia, especially women who menstruate heavily. Eating red meat more often, however, is not advisable because of the harmful saturated fats it contains, including large amounts of palmitic acid.

Eating lots of red meat can also cause colorectal cancer, one of the most common cancers in the West (as was seen among Asian immigrants in the United States who began to suffer high rates of colorectal cancer after switching from native diets to the beef-based diet of their new country). Other cancers that have been associated with too much red meat include stomach, throat, and breast cancer, although the link is weaker.

Accordingly, the best thing you can do in the meat section is to buy in moderation, in small portions, and choose lean meats. You don't have to forsake that beautifully marbled 300-gram steak altogether, just reserve it for special occasions.

When it comes to poultry, we can afford to be more generous. Since they have less saturated and more unsaturated fat than beef, chicken, turkey, and other poultry have a healthier fat profile and can be eaten several times a week. Breast meat is best, since it contains less fat than thighs or wings. The skin contains still more fat, so you will want to remove it before eating. To eliminate any possible trace of salmonella, cook poultry thoroughly: bacteria do not withstand heat well. And try to avoid the fried chicken from fast-food chains: although the fat profile of the chicken is fine, the trans fats used in the fryer is dynamite in your arteries.

Last stop: pork. In the form of chops or loin, pork lies halfway between red meat and poultry. Its fat profile is neither as negative as beef nor as positive as chicken; let's put it in the twice-a-week category.

Sausage, luncheon meats, and the like merit their own section because they contain much more fat and thus much more saturated fat than pork loin or chops. For example, 100 grams of sausage or bologna typically contain between 30 and 40 grams of fat, whereas 100 grams of loin contain just 10 grams of fat.

The fat profile depends on how the pig is raised. Free-range pigs feeding on acorns produce the delicious Jabugo hams of Spain, which, like olive oil, are rich in monounsaturated fats. At the other end of the spectrum, when pigs are raised on artificial feed on factory farms, levels of undesirable saturated fats in the meat soar. With prepared meats, such as sausages, the consumer has no way of knowing how they are even made, how much salt, or what fats, if any, are added, and what parts of the pig are used. And they may well comply with health laws. But such standards are aimed more at preventing food poisoning in the short term than at ensuring long-term health. So you would be wise to eat such meats in moderation.

Other Sources of Protein

Before you head for the checkout counter, pause for a moment in the nuts section. Here you find an assortment of delights as rich in protein as any of the meats you put in your basket. If 100 grams of beef tenderloin has about 20 grams of protein, 100 grams of peanuts has 25. After peanuts, nuts rank as follows: almonds (19 grams), pistachios (18), walnuts (15), and hazelnuts (12, though second in terms of monounsaturated fats, after Macadamia nuts). In addition to nuts, other plant products that contain protein include soybeans (no. 1 with 34 grams of protein per hundred grams of dry weight), spaghetti (4 grams after boiling), potatoes (2 grams), and even lettuce (1.3 grams, although lettuce is 95 percent water).

Actually, all plants contain protein. The problem, and it makes a big difference, is that the human body processes animal protein better than vegetable protein; since part of vegetable protein is lost without being absorbed, you have to eat more vegetables to get the amino acids your body needs. The second major difference is that plant proteins are low in biological value, meaning they do not provide all eight essential amino acids. Not that vegetable proteins are not good; it's just that they are not enough on their own unless you know how to balance your diet correctly to include plant products that provide the amino acids that are missing in others.

The one exception, the only plant that provides high biological value protein, is soybeans, which can provide as many essential proteins as meat, without boosting cholesterol. Not only that—if you get your protein from soy products such as tofu or soy milk, it will help lower your bad cholesterol and triglycerides while maintaining good cholesterol. Soybeans are also extraordinarily rich in isoflavones, which help prevent heart disease, some cancers such as breast and uterine cancer, and possibly osteoporosis. The benefits of soy are so clear that the U.S. Food and Drug Administration permits labeling of products with over 6.25 grams of soy protein per serving as heart-healthy.

To Be or Not to Be (a Vegetarian)? That Is the Question

So, going back to that patient who posited the idea of quitting meat to ward off the effects of age, there is no doubt that a vegetarian diet helps you stay healthy (Fig. 8).

"Not only that," I told him, "obesity, high cholesterol, and cardiovascular diseases are rare among vegetarians. But we do not know to what extent this is due to diet or to the fact that vegetarians tend to lead healthy lives in general."

Nor is there any doubt that a non-meat diet is no guarantee of good health. Cases of anemia due to lack of iron are not rare among vegetarians. The same for vitamin B_{12}, vitamin D, and calcium deficiencies. And, of course, I would not recommend a strict vegetarian diet for pregnant women or nursing mothers, or a child or teenager because any nutrient deficiency during growth can mark a child for the rest of his life.

"But if you want to keep fit and remain healthy," I continued, "it is not a question of being a vegetarian or not. It is a question of having a proper diet or not. Be a vegetarian if you like. But an ideal diet that includes meat and fish is also possible. You just have to ensure that you follow a varied diet, without too many calories, with lots of fruit and vegetables, low in saturated fats. And whatever you eat, make sure you get enough protein so your body can regenerate the millions of cells that die every day."

CHAPTER TWELVE

Carbohydrates

SWEETS THAT SOUR

We have lost respect for food. We have so much of it and it is so cheap and so easy to prepare—just remove the plastic, put the dish in the microwave for 2 minutes and abracadabra, dinner is served—that we scarcely give it a thought. The old ritual of the family gathered around the table enjoying a meal that someone actually put effort into preparing is now an anachronism in many homes, an exception reserved for special occasions: a birthday, a candlelight dinner with one's partner, Christmas Day. But in our busy daily life, we tend to do what's easiest, which usually means sitting in front of the TV and paying more attention to what is on the screen than on the plate. We don't eat; we ingest. Any time of the day. Which often leads to eating more, enjoying it less, and eating worse.

Take the example of carbohydrates. We eat fewer potatoes and chickpeas and more candy. That is, complex carbohydrates with high nutritive value are in decline, while sugars that provide instant gratification but have scarce nutritional value are on the rise.

This is what surveys show in Spain, for instance, per capita consumption of potatoes has fallen by around 17 percent in ten years; at the same time, consumption of sweets has increased, and now more than 40 percent of the Spanish population, children and adults, consume candy or chewing gum at least four times a week.

And one wonders: Why is all this happening? What causes these trends? It may have to do with the tight schedules and hurried lifestyle of urban societies. It's not only that we do not have time to make a nice pot of stewed chickpeas: It's also a matter of impatience, the rush for immediate pleasure, the sweetness of candy that offers a quick lift, much quicker than slow-digesting cereals and pulses.

Perhaps it is simply that most people like Dum Dums better than chickpeas. And if people like Dum Dums, one may wonder: What's wrong with eating them?

Rich Carbohydrate Food Examples

The numbers indicate the content, in grams, of the different nutrients for every 100 grams of food.

Complex Carbohydrates	Carbohydrates	Fats	Proteins
Bread (wheat)	48	1	8
Boiled potato	15	0	2
French fries	36	14	4
Egg pasta (boiled, with no sauce)	24	1	4
Rice (boiled, with no sauce)	20	0	2
Garbanzos	16	2	7
Breakfast cereal (Cornflakes, with no sugar)	86	0.5	8

Simple Carbohydrates	Carbohydrates	Fats	Proteins
Hard candy	88	0	0
Soft candy (like toffee)	68	18	2
Ice cream (vanilla)	24	10	4
Chocolate (dark, 60% cocao)	47	30	5
Custard	15	3	2.5
Honey	75	0	0.5
Commercial orange juice	9	0	0.5

Empty Calories

What is wrong with candy that it does not contain the same type of carbohydrate as vegetables and grains. Candy contains what we call simple carbohydrates, or sugars, which are digested quickly, go immediately into the blood, and provide energy, namely calories, but have no vitamins, minerals, or any other nutrients. That is why we call them empty calories—because they provide energy without nutrients.

Simple carbohydrates include sucrose (common sugar), fructose from fruit, lactose from milk, and glucose, the sugar your body makes from the food it digests and which is found in your blood.

Foods such as bread, pasta, potatoes, or rice, on the other hand, are rich in what we call complex carbohydrates. These are long chains of sugars that the digestive system must break down into simple carbohydrates in order to convert them into glucose and harness their energy. Like sugars, complex carbohydrates are fuel for the human body: they are not used to regenerate organs, as proteins are, but are used as an energy source.

But the foods that contain them are often vegetables rich in fiber, vitamins, minerals, and proteins: in other words, foods with much higher nutritional value than sweets. Another advantage of complex carbohydrates, especially for diabetics, is that, since we digest them slowly, unlike candy they do not cause the glucose in the blood to rise suddenly.

Fiber is also a carbohydrate, not because it provides calories but rather because of its chemical composition. In reality, fiber has a very different effect from that of other carbohydrates: instead of providing energy, it makes you feel full, which helps you limit your calorie intake. Other benefits of fiber, as we saw in chapter 9, are that it helps control blood sugar levels and blood cholesterol and it facilitates the passage of food through the intestinal tract.

From the Savanna to the Supermarket

Of course, all types of carbohydrates fit into a healthy diet. But because they must provide over half the calories in your diet, abundant daily intake of complex carbohydrates is recommended, whereras moderation is the rule with sugars.

However, for some reason we do not really understand, we seem to be wired the wrong way around so that we find sugars appetizing and complex carbohydrates such as boiled potatoes insipid. Perhaps that is because the sugars are high-octane fuel for the human body, the fastest way to get energy, and that the taste for sweet flavors is life insurance that evolution invented to prevent deaths from hypoglycemia, that is, from insufficient blood sugar.

In any case, what we do know is that our brain does not have an effective mechanism to regulate sugar consumption, so the point at which the brain says "I do not want more" is well above the limit of what is healthy. It is as if we were designed to avoid a shortage but not an excess of sugar.

This might have been reasonable a million years ago, when *Homo erectus* was chasing antelopes across the savanna, food was scarce, and a bounty of fructose was a guarantee of surviving until the next day. But it is a contradiction in present-day societies where we have access to more food than we need and where more people die from too many calories rather than from too few.

Bread, Potatoes, and Spaghetti

Another major contradiction is that some of the healthiest foods containing carbohydrates have such a bad reputation that many people avoid them, while other less healthy foods are eaten in massive quantities.

Bread, for example, is often singled out as fattening. And that is undeniably so: if you eat too much of it, bread is indeed fattening. But the problem is not bread itself but eating too much of it. Too much protein or too much fat is fattening, too. The same is true if you use bread to sop up sauce or eat it with cheese, sausage, or butter and jam.

But the problem in these cases is not the bread but the high-calorie foods you eat it with. Bread, as we see, is an innocent victim of the other foods we so often slather it with. And if you want to lose weight, you can moderate your consumption of sandwiches or toast-with-Nutella, but there is no justification for becoming so obsessed that you strike bread entirely from your diet.

The same goes for spaghetti or potatoes, which also have a reputation for being fattening and which some slimming diets ban—unfairly so because a plate of pasta or a grilled potato does not contain a prohibitive amount of calories. But if you eat pasta with a four-cheese sauce or eat your potatoes fried instead of baked, clearly the number of calories is going to shoot up. For those who like pasta but fear the calories in sauces, a good solution can be to season spaghetti with a bit of olive oil and seasonings such as oregano, black pepper, or basil.

The only valid criticism of white bread and potatoes is that they are digested within minutes and quickly raise glucose levels in the blood, not as much as candy but more than other foods with complex carbohydrates, such as lentils or pasta. But this increase in glucose is irrelevant if you eat two or three slices of bread or a potato with meals. In any case, if you are concerned about glucose, you can always eat whole grain bread, which has more fiber than white bread, and fiber slows glucose absorption. The truth is that low-carb slimming diets work no better than other diets.

Indeed, an ideal balanced diet, according to the American Heart Association, should be generous not low in carbohydrates. In the food pyramid that illustrates how much you should consume of different types of foods for an ideal diet, complex carbohydrates form the base, meaning that they should be eaten in the greatest quantities (see Fig. 8). And if the first of the ten recommendations of the panel of experts that reviewed the available scientific evidence on diet and cardiovascular disease was to "eat a variety of fruits and vegetables," the second recommendation is to "eat a variety of grain foods, including whole grains, at least six servings a day." A serving in this case equals 60 grams (2.1 ounces) of rice or pasta, potato, or half of a small roll.

Whole grains are especially recommended because they contain more fiber, more healthy fats, and more vitamins, minerals, and antioxidants than refined grains. It is not that refined grains are not good; it's just that whole grains are better. Different studies have found that the more whole foods you eat, the lower the risk of cardiovascular disease. Many of the benefits are attributed to the fiber in grains, which in terms of preventing cardiovascular disease has been shown to be even better than that in fruit and vegetables. But fiber is not enough to explain all the salutary effects seen among people who eat a lot of whole grains; some of the benefits must be due to the vitamins, minerals, antioxidants, and fats they contain. Complex carbohydrates, therefore, should be the mainstay of most meals.

The age-old idea of meat or fish as the most important part of a meal is, with all we know today about nutrition, passé. If you are going to make a meal of a single dish, as millions of people do when they are rushed, it is often better to make it rich in carbohydrates instead of proteins. And if you are having a side dish, a bit of meat with a lot of rice is better than the other way around.

Cakes and Dum Dums

With simple carbohydrates the story is the other way around. Although they are filled with empty calories and cause an abrupt rise in blood sugar, many people do not consider them harmful and see nothing wrong with eating them on a regular basis. That is the great paradox of carbohydrates: we worry about the healthier ones and we do not stop to think about the most worrisome ones.

I remember a patient who had started a diet and swore he was sticking to our recommendations, but he was not getting any thinner. He was telling the truth; he was following our advice. But talking with him, we discovered that what he drank most was Coca-Cola. He drank Coke every day—several times a day. It did not occur to him to tell us, and it did not occur to us to ask. He had not told us because he did not count Coke as food. It was a treat. But it was a treat that gave him an injection of a few hundred extra calories a day.

This problem, regularly consuming foods that should be consumed only occasionally, is the most common error people make with simple carbohydrates. It's not just Coca-Cola: it's candy, ice cream, cookies, fruit juices, all those products that fit into a *weekly* balanced diet but have found a place in the *daily* diet.

Moreover, they tend to displace other foods that should get top billing in a daily diet but are now relegated to occasional consumption. A perfect example are sugary desserts. Cakes, ice cream, custard, chocolate pudding, milk shakes. . . the list is endless. Can they be part of a healthy diet? Undoubtedly. Can you eat them every day?

A defense lawyer might argue yes: they are high in nutritional value, in general thanks to the proteins they contain; they are good for a child's development; they taste good; some come in low-fat versions that do not create cholesterol problems.

A prosecutor might object that sugary desserts tend to be high in empty calories; others try to pass themselves off as healthy when in fact they contain high amounts of sugars or fats; others claim, but do not demonstrate, that they stimulate the immune system.

Yet the worst part of putting sweet desserts on the daily menu is the collateral damage to fruit consumption: the more sweet desserts, the less fruit and, hence, less fiber, less vitamins, less antioxidants. Less health.

Moreover, when there are children in the household, putting sweets before fruit sets a poor example and teaches them to see fruit as being dispensable, rather than to appreciate it as a staple food in a healthy diet. The same goes for candy. Or cookies.

The problem is not that the sugar in a Dum Dums or four Starbursts is going to destroy your child's health. Generally speaking, it will not, except for the risk of cavities. The problem is that when children are allowed to eat sweets on a daily basis, as happens in almost half the households in Spain, it is unlikely that they are being taught to eat right.

Rather than let your child have a lollipop or chew gum when they want, personally, I think it is worthwhile to try to teach children from an early age that there are foods that should be eaten every day, such as fruit or milk, and others, such as candy, that are very tasty but should be eaten only occasionally.

Overweight and Diabetes

And it's not that I do not like sweets. On the contrary, I love them. If I had followed my instincts, I would have become a pastry chef.

But what usually happens when you eat a lot of simple carbohydrates in the form of candy is that you end up getting too many calories. And that is because people so often eat candy— on the run, out of the vending machine—in addition to, rather than instead of, other foods. Candy is, like Coke for that patient of mine, a treat. A treat that eventually ends up as a few extra pounds, then higher cholesterol, higher blood pressure, and—as demonstrated in a study of the links between diet and health in more than 75,000 women over ten years—greater risk of coronary disease. So, in its dietary guidelines, the American Heart Association expressly recommends limiting high-calorie and nutritionally poor foods, including soft drinks and candy with a lot of sugar.

On the other hand, and contrary to widespread belief, sweets do not have a direct impact on the risk of developing diabetes.

They have an indirect impact since too many calories lead to overweight, and overweight is directly associated with risk of diabetes. But the most common cause of diabetes is not too much sugar in the diet but excess fat in the abdomen, which in many cases is not related to a diet rich in sugary foods.

The confusion arises because diabetes is a breakdown in the body's ability to keep its blood sugar levels under control. But it is wrong to make what may seem the obvious association: that if you have too much sugar in your diet, you will get excess blood sugar. It is true that, right after eating sugary foods, blood glucose rises. But it is a transitory effect, normal in healthy people, and has nothing to do with diabetes.

In fact, there are two different types of diabetes. What we call Type 1 diabetes, less common but more serious, usually appears during childhood by destroying cells in the pancreas that produce insulin, the hormone that regulates blood sugar. Type 2 diabetes, which affects nearly 15 million people in the United States, often appears in adults because abdominal fat secretes substances that interfere with the action of insulin.

Although carbohydrates do not have a big impact on the origin of diabetes, they do have a big impact on the disease once it has developed. Since their insulin is out of whack, people with diabetes suffer a sharp rise in blood glucose every time they eat starches or carbohydrates. This excess glucose damages arteries, which facilitates cholesterol deposits and the advance of atherosclerosis. Excessive levels of glucose also promote blood inflammation, increasing the risk of clotting, and, in overweight people, causes high blood pressure, increases bad cholesterol, lowers good cholesterol, increases triglycerides—in short, an all-out attack on the heart and arteries.

That's why it's so important to check your blood glucose after forty-five years of age: check it every three years, ensuring that it does not exceed 100 mg/dl after fasting, for early detection of a prediabetic condition, and to take action before it can wreak havoc on your arteries.

The measures taken in cases of Type 2 diabetes, the most common form, start with diet. People with Type 1 diabetes, which destroys pancreatic cells, must rely on insulin injections from the outset. But with Type 2, when the pancreas secretes insulin but this insulin does not manage to control blood glucose, the first thing the patient should do is lose weight. The idea is to reduce the amount of abdominal fat, and thus the production of substances that interfere with insulin; the hope is that insulin will regain its ability to regulate glucose levels.

This is a stage where diabetes is still reversible. Hence the importance of early diagnosis and strict diet: if we do not control the disease from the outset, when there is still time, the subsequent damage cannot be undone.

People with diabetes can eat the same things that a healthy person does, provided that the healthy person has a proper diet. But if you have diabetes you should be especially careful to avoid high or low blood glucose. Thus, it is better to shun sugary foods and eat lots of fiber, since fiber slows sugar absorption and helps prevent spikes in glucose levels. Although all fiber-rich foods are recommended, studies with diabetic patients have shown that barley, oats, rye, and whole wheat pasta are particularly effective.

The irony of it all is that so often it is only when one falls sick that one discovers the wonders of a healthy diet—not only with diabetes but with many diseases.

Nor is it true that negligent diet explains all cases of diabetes, cardiovascular diseases, or digestive disorders. I have seen many patients who have always eaten well but fell sick nonetheless.

But I have seen many more who only started to care the day they got sick. And perhaps had they worried just a bit more about what they ate from the outset, they would not have so much to worry about now.

CHAPTER THIRTEEN

Alcohol

IN PRAISE OF MODERATION

"I'm doing the right thing, aren't I, Doctor? I drink wine every day."

It is a typical question. A lot of patients ask the same thing. And the typical response is: "No, you're not doing the right thing, not at all, drinking as much as you do."

"But I thought wine was good for your heart."

"Wine can be good for your heart, but it can also be bad for your heart and for your body. It all depends on how much and how you drink."

What happens in most patients is that the damage from alcohol far outweighs the benefits. In theory, it is true that wine and other alcoholic beverages may be beneficial to cardiovascular health. But I recommend that my patients not drink more alcohol but less.

I see so many people who believe they are doing something healthy when in reality they are doing something harmful. This is an example of how a misconception can spread like an epidemic. Because what we have is a real epidemic of misunderstanding about alcohol.

Benefits of Moderate Consumption

But let's start with the good news. Some studies have shown that moderate intake of alcohol, equivalent to one or two glasses of wine a day, may reduce the risk of cardiovascular disease up to 15 percent, which is an incredible rate. In people who are already ill, it may also reduce mortality up to 15 percent. A drug so effective, i.e., that prevented one or two out of every ten deaths from cardiovascular diseases, would be an extraordinary breakthrough. But the fact is, if in addition to having the same effectiveness as wine, the drug had the same risks associated with overdose, the government would not authorize its sale.

The benefits of a daily glass of wine became part of popular lore in the 1980s when people started talking about the French paradox. The paradox was that in France, where the consumption of saturated fats was similar to the United States, there were far lower rates of coronary disease. If saturated fats are the key to cardiovascular risk, where did the difference lie?

Part of this phenomenon can be explained by the fact that the French eat more fruits and vegetables. But the difference was so vast that there had to be another factor. That other factor, it was thought, might be wine.

More recent studies have confirmed that wine actually does protect the heart and arteries. Wine, it was discovered, acts as a powerful anticoagulant, comparable to aspirin. It seems that it inhibits clotting in several ways at once: on the one hand, it inhibits the action of platelets, tiny components of the blood (there are 250 million in each cubic centimeter) specialized in forming clots; it reduces the production of fibrinogen, a protein necessary to clotting; and it reduces the production of tissue factor, another coagulant protein.

For the anticoagulant effects alone, one or two glasses of wine a day would be beneficial to cardiovascular health. But wine is also a powerful anti-inflammatory, it can reduce levels of C-reactive protein in the blood and inhibit monocytes in the immune system so that they do not trigger a heart attack. It's good for managing fats, since it can increase HDL, good cholesterol, by no less than 12 percent. It helps you manage your sugar by enhancing the effectiveness of insulin in regulating blood glucose. And it contains antioxidants, although we do not know how large an impact these substances have on preventing cardiovascular accidents. If wine was not so problematic otherwise, it would be a health wonder.

All these benefits not only prevent heart attacks but they also lower the risk of cerebral vascular accidents like stroke. And the risk of peripheral vascular disease, in which the problems of blood flow to the legs make something as simple as walking excruciatingly painful, also decreases with moderate consumption of wine.

On the other hand, it has yet to be demonstrated that wine is of any use in preventing any type of cancer. It has been discovered that red wine contains a substance, resveratrol, that under laboratory conditions inhibits the proliferation of cancer cells. But the human body is an infinitely more complex system than cells cultivated in a lab and no study has demonstrated that the resveratrol in wine reduces the risk of cancer or has any benefits for a patient diagnosed with a tumor. In fact, recent studies have opened the possibility that wine may contribute to some kinds of cancer.

Wine or Beer?

As we learn more about how alcoholic beverages affect cardiovascular health, we have discovered that their main benefits are not due to components specific to red wine, such as tannins or resveratrol, but to the alcohol itself. In the late 1980s and 1990s people were talking mainly about red wine because, after the discovery of the French paradox, it was the focus of early studies.

But since then we have come to realize that the main benefits of moderate wine intake are mainly due to the alcohol, which is where it gets its strong anticoagulant and anti-inflammatory effects, and thus these effects are common to all alcoholic beverages. Perhaps other benefits such as antioxidant and vasodilator effects are specific to red wine because they are due not to alcohol but to other substances. But these benefits seem minor compared to the direct action of alcohol.

So when someone asks me what sort of wine is best for the heart, I say:

"Look, so long as you drink it in moderation, drink whichever type you like. Your heart doesn't care if you drink red, white, or rosé, or champagne, or even beer. But if you are not going to drink it in moderation, it is better not to drink it at all."

As far as your heart is concerned, whether the alcohol comes from a snifter of cognac or a shot of rum, the effect is the same. If no one defends the cardiovascular benefits of high-proof drinks, it is not because the alcohol they contain is worse, but because they are not often associated with moderation: people who finish off a meal with a whiskey or brandy are likely to already have half a bottle of wine under their belt.

How Much Should I Drink?

Now that we have enjoyed our one or two glasses of wine, I would add that I personally do not advise anyone to drink alcohol for health reasons. And I do not make such recommendations because they raise questions that doctors have yet to resolve.

The first question is how to ensure that people drink only enough to get the benefits and not so much that the alcohol harms them. If human beings were perfectly rational, it would be easy. It would be enough to explain that you get the maximum benefits with one drink a day for women and two a day for men. And that a drink means 10 grams of alcohol, which is roughly the amount in a glass of wine or small glass of beer. For people who would like to know exactly how much alcohol they ingest, it is not difficult to calculate.

If a beer is 5 percent alcohol, this means that for every 100 grams (or 100 cubic centimeters) you drink, you get 5 grams of alcohol. Thus, the 20 grams of alcohol a day recommended for a man is equivalent to 400 cubic centimeters (6.7 ounces) of beer.

The same goes for wine: if it is 12 percent alcohol, for every hundred grams of wine, roughly 12 are alcohol. Therefore, a standard 75 cL-bottle of wine contains about 90 grams of pure alcohol, and a man would then get his recommended 20 grams a day from 170 cubic centimeters (5.7 ounces), which amounts to two glasses of wine.

You should also know that in order to enjoy the health benefits of alcohol, you must drink the recommended amount every day, not abstain for six days and then polish off an entire bottle on Saturday night. That would be like taking seven aspirins on Saturday after not having taken any for a week: you lose all the advantages of daily moderate consumption and get all the harm of a Saturday night binge.

With these simple guidelines in mind, if people were more prone to rational behavior, we could all enjoy the virtues of alcoholic beverages and we'd see a major drop in the rate of cardiovascular disease. But in real life most people do not behave like that. Everyone has their own problems, their own contradictions, their silent inner battle between reason and emotion. And the end result of all this unconscious conflict in the brain is that when a doctor tells a patient he can have two drinks a day, the patient will probably end up having four.

At four drinks a day, we are no longer talking about healthy intake, but nor have we yet reached the point of alcoholism. We have reached a stage we call risky consumption, which is the anteroom to misfortune. An at-risk drinker does not have problems stemming from alcohol, but he probably will in the future. For men, risky consumption is generally considered to start at 40 grams of alcohol a day, equivalent to 2.5 cans of beer or a half-bottle of wine. For women, the threshold of risk is 25 grams of alcohol a day, equivalent to half a liter (17 ounces) of beer or two glasses of wine.

How to Calculate Your Alcohol Intake

About 20 grams of alcohol a day for men and 10 grams for women is appropriate. From 40 grams of alcohol a day for males and 25 for females, the risks outweigh the benefits. To calculate how much alcohol you drink, the following equivalencies may be useful:

	Percent	Volume	Grams of Alcohol
Beer	5%	small glass 200 ml	10 g
		can 320 ml	16 g
Wine	12%	100 ml	12 g
Sherry or similar	20%	50 ml	10 g
Distillates	40%	shot 25 ml	10 g
		glass or mixed drink 50 ml	20 g

Different People, Different Effects

These amounts, 40 grams as an upper limit for men and 25 grams for women, are only guidelines. In reality—this is the second major question we face in recommending consumption of wine or beer—the response to alcohol varies enormously from one person to another.

To begin with, it varies between men and women because men tend to have a larger quantity of a substance that metabolizes alcohol in the liver. Therefore, when a man and woman share a bottle of wine, after dinner there is usually a higher concentration of alcohol in the woman's blood than in the man's. Which is precisely why the thresholds for optimal and risky consumption are lower for women.

Even within the male or female population, alcohol can affect different people very differently. Common sense tells us that a man who weighs 90 kilograms (198 pounds) can, in principle, tolerate a greater quantity of alcohol than another weighing 60 kilograms (132 pounds). But weight is not the only factor; it is not even the most important factor. We know that there are people who drink a lot and never have major alcohol-related problems, while others start to have problems when they drink only a little. And if the harmful effects of alcohol vary according to the person, odds are the beneficial effects also vary.

We do not yet know what causes these differences, but a similar phenomenon occurs with aspirin. For reasons not well understood, aspirin is very effective for preventing heart attacks in 25 percent of the population, while the remaining 75 percent for whatever reason is less responsive. And since we do not understand why this happens, you have no way of knowing to what extent alcohol is good for you, what the optimal dose is for you, or at what point you cross the line to become an at-risk drinker.

It is a mistake to think that because it might not go to your head, alcohol does not affect you and thus you can tolerate greater amounts. Because one thing is what happens in the brain, which tends to adjust to larger and larger doses of any drug (which is why the occasional drinker often feels tipsy after the first beer, while a regular drinker may not feel a thing after the fourth).

What happens in the rest of your body, where alcohol affects many organs, is another question altogether. So you might think there's no harm in a glass of cognac after wine with dinner and a beer to kick the evening off because your brain is so used to alcohol that it does not feel the slightest effect. But meanwhile other, more selfless organs—your liver, pancreas, and even your heart—suffer the ravages of alcohol in silence. We see, then, that the effects of alcohol not only vary from one person to another but from one organ to another.

A third question we face in making recommendations regarding alcohol is that the optimal dose to protect the heart is different from the optimal dose to protect the brain. If we want to prevent heart disease and thus death from heart attack, 10 grams of alcohol a day (a glass of wine or small beer) is ideal for a man. But if we want to prevent stroke, the ideal level appears to be larger.

There are so many unknowns about alcohol that the only thing we can say without fear of causing anyone harm is that a glass of wine a day for women (10 grams of alcohol) and two glasses for men (20 grams) is appropriate. That does not mean these are the best possible levels for everyone. But they are cautious levels that appear to be beneficial to almost everyone, the big exception being recovering alcoholics, for whom not even a daily glass of wine is recommended.

Above these levels, in the range of 10 grams of alcohol a day for women and 20 grams for men, the picture goes fuzzy. We know from epidemiological studies on alcohol and health that such levels are good for some people and bad for others, but since we have no way of knowing who wins and who loses, we do not recommend them.

Above 20 grams a day for women and 40 for men, there is no doubt that the harm outweighs the benefits.

Another Drink, Another Risk

One of the most significant effects of alcohol abuse, and one that goes largely unnoticed, is obesity. Each gram of alcohol provides seven calories, almost twice as much as a gram of sugar or meat. So, every can of beer you drink contains over 100 calories, which is equivalent to a 100-gram (3.5 ounces) steak. And when you exceed 40 grams of alcohol a day, you are taking in over 280 extra calories. So when an overweight or obese person moderates their alcohol consumption—for example, drinking water instead of wine with meals—they achieve weight loss that is significant and lasting.

In people with hypertension, drinking less lowers blood pressure to safer levels. Research shows that for women who have over two drinks a day and men who have over four, maximum pressure rises by ten millimeters of mercury and minimum by five. After the fourth drink for women and the sixth for men, the risk of brain hemorrhage due to hypertension increases.

So one of the first recommendations for a person diagnosed with hypertension is not to drink alcohol. If you keep hypertension under control, for example with diet, physical activity, and drugs, you can have one or two drinks a day without fear of ending up in the hospital. But no more than one or two because once you cross that line, even by a little, alcohol stops preventing stroke and starts causing it.

With what we know about the impact of alcohol on obesity and blood pressure, we cannot say that alcohol is good for the heart and bad for other organs, as all those patients proud of their daily wine drinking believe. This interpretation is simplistic and misleading because, for the heart, too, wine can be harmful.

We know that alcohol abuse raises the level of undesirable triglycerides in the blood. We know that it triggers arrhythmias and causes sudden death, and it does so without the need to get drunk: sustained high consumption, one day after another, is enough. We know that it contributes to dilated cardiomyopathy, a condition where the heart becomes enlarged and cannot pump blood efficiently.

And for other organs the picture is no prettier. Alcohol abuse leads to cirrhosis of the liver; to pancreatitis in the pancreas; to myopathies in the muscles. It leads to addiction, and alcoholism is a particularly devastating addiction in the brain. It leads to depressive psychiatric disorders and to anxiety disorders. And, apparently, it may lead to a panoply of cancers: mouth, pharynx, larynx, esophagus, liver, breast, and colorectal.

To give an example of the impact of alcohol on the population of a country: according to data from the Spanish National Statistical Institute, one out of every fifteen deaths in Spain is directly attributable to alcohol abuse. And contrary to widespread belief, the problem affects the female population just as much as the male.

There is a misperception that alcohol abuse is much more prevalent among men than women. But at the hospital, what we find is that when a man with a drinking problem is admitted, he usually says so, but when it is a woman in the same situation, she usually hides it. She may hide her problem so well that not even her family is aware. And surely this happens because we live in a society where alcohol abuse in men is accepted, even admired, while in women it is frowned upon, which drives many women to drink in secret.

Basic Recommendations

Given this scenario, what recommendations can doctors give regarding alcohol? The risk of being misunderstood is so great—as evidenced by all the patients who think they are doing the right thing when the truth is they are drinking more than they should—that I believe we should not encourage anyone to drink more than they already do.

If someone does not drink, they should continue to not drink. This is particularly important among young people since if you promote moderate drinking among twenty- or twenty-five-year-olds, you may be promoting alcoholism in their forties. If someone has one or two drinks a day, the best thing they can do is not change their ways. And if they are having more than three drinks, which is a case I often see, the best thing we can do is advise them to cut down to one or two.

"But I feel fine," a friend told me one day. "And I like to drink wine with meals."

Between lunch and dinner he was drinking about a bottle a day. I told him what 90 grams of alcohol a day does to your body in the long term, and I let him decide whether to go on like that or cut back. He decided not to cut back. In summer 2005, while on vacation, I received a call from him. He had landed in the emergency room with an arrhythmia.

CHAPTER FOURTEEN

Tobacco

HOW TO QUIT SMOKING

The best way to quit smoking is to have a heart attack. We see it every day at the hospital, and a multitude of studies have confirmed it. People smoke for decades, knowing that tobacco is harmful, telling themselves someday they will have to quit but never making any serious attempt. Then the day they have a heart attack and start to really fear for their lives, they say that's it.

Like the man who smoked two packs a day and shrugged it off saying that his father smoked until the age of ninty-five and died of a fractured femur. Like the woman who did not try to quit because she was afraid she would put on weight. And another woman who had tried nicotine gum, patches, and acupuncture and always slid back into smoking. All of these are real cases involving real people I've come across in the past six months.

I've been seeing these cases, identical stories involving different people, for over thirty years. And what usually happens in the end is that when you realize that your life is at stake, the fact that your father smoked until he was ninety-five or that you might gain a few pounds no longer matters. That day, when you find yourself in the hospital after a bypass operation, you feel motivated to at least try to quit.

Few people succeed at first. Beating an addiction is not easy for anyone, and over half of those who try to quit start smoking again within a year. But relapse need not be seen as failure. Instead, I see it as a breakthrough because a smoker who tries and fails is more likely to succeed the second time than one who has never tried before. And if you fail again, the statistics show that you are more likely than not to succeed on the third attempt. In the end, although it is not easy for anyone, anyone can quit if they want to. That is the key: wanting to.

The Ravages of Tobacco

With tobacco, we do not have the same blurred lines as with alcohol, which may be healthy in small amounts and harmful in high amounts: smoking is harmful from the first cigarette.

First of all, tobacco triggers your entire blood clotting system, and so increases the risk of clotting and thus the risk of stroke and heart attack. This is an immediate effect of tobacco and that's why when you stop smoking, the risk of a cardiovascular accident falls after a few weeks. So the benefits of quitting are also immediate.

Moreover, the thousands of toxic components in tobacco smoke cause chronic damage to the tissues it comes into contact with. In your lungs, it causes cell mutations that can lead to cancer. It causes chronic obstructive pulmonary disease (COPD), an irreversible condition, which is characterized by shortness of breath and is the leading cause of respiratory death. Smoking also causes cancer of the mouth, larynx, esophagus, stomach, bladder, kidney, and pancreas. All of these are long-term effects, which is why there are people who are diagnosed with lung cancer years after quitting: by the time they stopped smoking the transformation of cells toward cancer or the cancer itself might already have begun to develop.

All of these harmful effects occur with all forms of smoking tobacco, whether it is normal cigarettes, low tar cigarettes, and even cigars or a pipe. I have heard people say that smoking cigars is not as harmful as smoking cigarettes, but the studies we have of cigar smokers belie that myth. Which is hardly surprising because the toxic elements in tobacco are there no matter how you smoke it. Blaming cigarettes and excusing cigars would be as absurd as claiming that canned beer gets you drunk and bottled does not.

Finally, as for the overall impact of smoking on health, the numbers speak for themselves: half of all smokers die prematurely from tobacco-related diseases. Today, tobacco kills more men than women, not because men are more vulnerable but because thirty years ago few women smoked. In the coming years, as more women who started smoking in the 1970s and '80s reach ages at which cancer and cardiovascular disease become more frequent, inevitably the death rate from tobacco will increase among the female population.

Are the Risks of Passive Smoking Exaggerated?

Many people in most countries, out of politeness, out of custom, or simply out of ignorance, continue to accept passive smoking. Although secondhand smoke bothers them, they rarely think it might be detrimental to their health. It is perceived as a nuisance rather than as a danger.

But after the effects of passive smoking on health were studied, it was found that it does not require large amounts of smoke to cause a significant impact on the blood. Simply having someone smoking next to you increases the risk of both clotting and what we call vasoconstriction, that is, a narrowing of the blood vessels. The effect is similar to that caused by spikes in air pollution levels. It is thought that the small particles inhaled probably increase the tendency for clots to form. A healthy person can handle these situations without suffering any appreciable harm. But for people who already have a coronary condition, passive smoke can trigger a heart attack.

The dangers of passive smoking have turned out to be greater than was thought a few years ago. The World Health Organization (WHO) has estimated that living with a smoker increases the risk of heart attack by 25 percent and the risk of lung cancer by 26 percent. In the United States it has been estimated that each year about four thousand people die from lung cancer due to passive smoking.

Bearing in mind the amount of smoke inhaled by a passive smoker, which is relatively small compared with an active smoker, these figures are far higher than what most people would have guessed. But the smoke that the active smoker inhales—what we call mainstream smoke—has a different composition from the smoke from the tip of the cigarette—secondary stream smoke. And this secondary stream, which is the only smoke inhaled by the passive smoker, has a higher concentration of some of the most toxic substances in tobacco.

Intrauterine Smoking

Particularly serious are the consequences of passive smoking in children. Because they breathe faster than adults and their bodies are smaller, children inhale more toxic waste per kilogram of weight. In addition, since their immune system is less developed, the younger the child the more prone they will be to respiratory infections caused by the toxins in tobacco smoke. The smoke itself does not cause infection; rather it makes the lungs more vulnerable to viruses and bacteria. According to WHO estimates, children of smoking mothers run a 70 percent higher risk of getting bronchitis. The risks of ear infection and asthma rise by near 50 percent when both parents smoke. And the risk of sudden infant death, when a newborn dies in his sleep without apparent cause, increases twofold in smoking households and sevenfold when the mother smokes more than one pack a day. In the United States, it has been estimated that more than two hundred children under one year of age die every year as victims of passive smoking.

And among intrauterine smokers, children whose mothers smoked or worked in a smoke-filled environment during pregnancy, there is a higher risk of low birth weight, which in turn increases the risk of infectious diseases, learning disabilities, and attention deficit disorder and hyperactivity during childhood. Which is why pregnancy is one of the best times to quit, since many mothers are willing to make sacrifices for their children that they would not make for themselves.

How to Quit: Set a Date and Seek Help

For people who want to quit smoking, in the absence of a specially strong motivation such as pregnancy or a heart attack, it is recommended that you start by setting a date. It may be New Year's Day, it may be your birthday or, better still, the birthday of your spouse (what better gift?), or it may be tomorrow.

But it is important to circle a date on the calendar—otherwise people always tend to leave it for next week—and look for a time when you feel emotionally stable. If you are going through a rough patch in your life, you are not likely to hold out long without smoking. So it's better to wait a few weeks or months for your prospects to improve.

Ideally, you should set the date in consultation with your doctor, rather than marking it on the kitchen calendar without anyone else knowing. There is no point in going to the doctor if you are not determined to quit because the doctor cannot quit for you. But if you have the motivation, you will have a better chance of succeeding if you seek help.

There are two types of therapy that have proved effective: counseling and treatment with drugs, of which the most common are nicotine chewing gum and patches. The highest rates of success are found where both types of treatments are combined.

Counseling helps the smoker identify stimuli, like coffee after a meal, that trigger the urge to light up, and provides strategies for breaking the link between smoking and those stimuli. At the same time, counseling includes techniques for dealing with stress and controlling situations that may lead to a relapse. You needn't go to the doctor often for psychological counseling to be effective. Telephone counseling, which permits more frequent contact between the doctor or nurse and the patient, can work even better.

Nicotine Patches or Gum?

Drug therapy, on the other hand, is intended to combat the nicotine withdrawal symptoms. These vary from one person to another but usually include irritability, anxiety, sadness, insomnia, difficulty concentrating, and increased appetite. We have two types of drugs that help overcome tobacco addiction: nicotine substitutes and an antidepressant.

Among nicotine substitutes, smokers have the choice between patches, chewing gum, or nasal inhalers. They are all equal in terms of effectiveness, and the choice depends on the preferences of the smoker. Patches have the advantages of being unobtrusive, easy to use, and delivering nicotine on an ongoing basis through the skin, so that the concentration of nicotine derivatives in the blood never falls. Gum and inhalers have the advantage of providing high doses of nicotine intermittently, which is closer to the actual effect of cigarettes. Although they are equally effective, more patients actually succeed in quitting with chewing gum or patches, probably because the inhalers are less discreet and less comfortable.

As for antidepressants, the only thing that is marketed as a treatment of smoking is bupropion. We do not have enough data to know whether it is more or less effective than nicotine substitutes. Nor is it clear whether combining the two treatments is more effective than either bupropion or nicotine alone.

Does Acupuncture Work?

No treatment, apart from counseling and drugs, has been proved to be an effective aid to quitting. Although some people have managed to quit smoking after trying acupuncture, clinical trials that have thoroughly examined the effects of acupuncture on smokers have failed to turn up evidence of its being more effective than no treatment at all.

Perhaps what happens here is that acupuncture, like drugs, works better with people who believe in it than with skeptics. My personal opinion is that acupuncture does little good because it does not force the person who wants to quit to take responsibility for his health. It's the same with dieting and what we said about people who put themselves in the hands of a dietitian but do not make a personal commitment to losing weight— they fail in the long term.

So, when a patient says they want to try acupuncture to quit smoking, I say: "Why not? It might work."

But if they do not mention it, I do not suggest it.

In situations like this, I believe that doctors should respect the freedom of each patient to do what they believe is best for themselves. Nicotine withdrawal involves anxiety, and everyone knows, generally better than their doctor, what their anxiety is like, what sparks it and how to cope with it. So if a person says that acupuncture works for them, I do not think there is any reason to discourage them. Other people prefer to carry around mints to ward off the withdrawal symptoms when the urge for a cigarette strikes, and that's fine. Still others prefer a glass of water, and that works for them. You know what is best for yourself.

Cold Turkey or Gradually?

Precisely because personal factors are so important, the best strategy for quitting smoking varies from one person to another. It varies according to the person's nature and the environment they live in.

What works best for people with the motivation and will-power is to quit cold: going from a pack or whatever you smoke a day to zero overnight. This method is common among people who have just suffered a heart attack; people that have resolved a personal conflict and are embarking on a new stage in life; and people who reach the conclusion that smoking is ruining their health.

I remember the case of a farmer from a village in Catalonia. He went to the doctor with a bad cough and the doctor told him that smoking was to blame. He had smoked for forty years without knowing that it was bad for him. And when he found out, he said, "That's it. I'm finished. I quit—starting this very moment."

The next morning, as he was going out to work in the fields, his wife was surprised to see him put a pack of cigarettes in his shirt pocket.

"Didn't you say you'd never smoke again?" she reproached him.

"And I won't. But I want to keep a pack on me because if I don't smoke, it'll be because I don't want to, not because I can't."

When he came home that evening, there was still the same number of cigarettes in the pack. For six months, every morning he went out with the pack in his pocket and came home without having smoked a single cigarette. Until one day, as he left for the fields, his wife remarked: "Alfons, you forgot your cigarettes."

"I don't need them anymore," he replied. He had quit on the strength of sheer willpower.

Cases like this, where motivation and willpower come together, have the best chance of success. At the other end of the spectrum we have a majority of smokers who more or less want to quit. They wish they had not started smoking in their youth but have neither the motivation nor the willpower they need to go cold turkey.

One strategy that works well with these smokers is to go out every morning with the exact number of cigarettes you are going to smoke that day. Then, every week you put in one fewer cigarette. What usually happens in the long term is that people get stuck at around half a pack a day. Since the risk of tobacco depends on the number of cigarettes you smoke, risk is reduced— not to zero but significantly. And if you are willing to further reduce the number of cigarettes you smoke, you may try cutting one cigarette every two weeks or every month with a six-month target of fewer than five per day.

The Partner Factor

Whether you go cold turkey or cut back week by week, it is often helpful to have the support of your partner or some other person you are close to. We have found that when a smoker is aware that their partner cares, they will usually try to quit. Similarly, smokers whose partners do not care, or care but do not say so, are less likely to quit.

If both people in a relationship smoke, it is almost impossible for either to quit on their own because they create a dynamic in which they smoke at the same times, share cigarettes, and may even use tobacco, albeit inadvertently, as a bonding mechanism. What works very well in these cases is for both smokers to try to quit at the same time.

If you do not have a partner to quit with, you can make a deal to quit at the same time with a friend or someone else you are close to. The mutual support of two people going through the same challenge and the desire not to fail each other, ease the pains of quitting and reduce the risk of relapse in the first few weeks.

On the other hand, support from your spouse, or whoever, is less effective when it is based on threats ("if you don't quit, it'll kill you") or recrimination ("you're a fool to start again, just when you'd managed to quit"). Rather, for both quitting and for the relationship, support based on positive attitudes ("I want you to quit because I care about your health") works better.

Do You Gain Weight When You Quit?

Despite all the benefits, quitting smoking has its drawbacks. Which is precisely why it is so hard to kick the habit. In the short term, all you get are the drawbacks; the rewards only come much later. Withdrawal starts a few hours after the last cigarette, hitting the peak of discomfort and bad temper between two and three days later, after which it fades slowly, taking weeks or months to disappear. The great merit of nicotine substitutes or bupropion, which are usually taken for two to six months, is that they alleviate withdrawal symptoms, which are temporary.

What is not usually temporary is the weight many smokers gain when they quit. One of the many effects of nicotine is that it inhibits appetite, so that smokers tend to eat fewer calories than non-smokers. In addition, they burn more calories because of the way tobacco affects their metabolism. These slimming effects of cigarettes disappear as soon as you quit. If we add the anxiety of withdrawal, which can lead to eating more, putting on seven or eight pounds is not uncommon for quitters.

Now, forget for a moment everything we said in previous chapters about how detrimental overweight is: those seven or eight pounds are the best investment a smoker can make in his or her health. A large number of women, as found in several studies, are reluctant to quit precisely because they are afraid they will put on weight, which is understandable. But it is ironic that they smoke to preserve their beauty when it causes premature aging of their skin and other organs.

So rather than continue smoking in order to keep your figure, the best thing you can do to protect your health and your beauty is to take steps to avoid weight gain when you quit smoking. One possibility is bupropion, which has been shown to have some effectiveness in controlling weight gain during withdrawal. But even more effective than bupropion is regular exercise. And not only because of the calories you burn but also because physical activity releases endorphins in the brain that act as an antidote to anxiety, and anxiety is one of the reasons why people tend to eat more when they stop smoking. And people who exercise tend to be more successful in quitting because they tend to be the sort of people who are more responsible about their health.

How to Avoid Backsliding

Even if you do everything right—set a day to quit and get counseling, exercise, and family support—one day you may still start smoking again. Among people who quit after having a heart attack, even with that motivation, plus support from their doctor and in most cases their family, over half start smoking again after a year. Studies of people who try patches show a success rate of nearly 30 percent. But this does not mean the remaining 70 percent will never kick the habit. It means that if they try again, another 28 percent will succeed on the second attempt. And other studies show that most smokers manage to quit in the first three attempts.

Nevertheless, the risk of backsliding always remains, and any ex-smoker can someday run into a situation they cannot handle. Everyone has a bad time of it some time in their life. What can be done in these cases is to try to control situations that may lead to that fateful first cigarette after months or years of abstinence:

situations such as a dinner with friends who smoke, or drinking a bit too much, since alcohol is a great uninhibitor and soon has you saying "one little cigarette isn't going to hurt me." But before having that first cigarette, remember that the ex-smoker who can smoke one cigarette, just one, and not get hooked again is the exception: most are back up to a pack within a month.

CHAPTER FIFTEEN

Exercise, Part 1

HOW TO GET STARTED ...

From the time the first humans appeared on Earth 2.5 million years ago, and for 99 percent of their existence thereafter, they led a nomadic life that entailed a great deal of physical activity. Only since agriculture and animal husbandry appeared about 10,000 years ago—when we gave up the uncertainty of mammoth hunts, foraging for berries in the forest, pulling up stakes and moving on to a new home every few weeks or months—have we enjoyed the tranquillity of a sedentary life, a period that covers just 0.4 percent of human history. And only in the last hundred years, or 0.004 percent of our history, with the invention of the lightbulb, the car, the elevator, central heating, the remote for your TV, and so many other laborsaving devices, have we reached an unprecedented level of physical inactivity and comfort. No other animal species needs to make so little effort to survive as a twenty-first-century human being.

But our body retains its memory of that 99.6 percent of human history when we still had to run every day in order to survive until the next. You only need to see the wondrous design of the human foot, with the front wider than the back for maximum propulsion with each stride, with its complex mechanism of perfectly articulated bones designed to optimize the transmission of energy from the heel to the tip—a machine built to run. Or watch children on the playground, how they run, jump, chase each other, shout. Or observe what the human body does when it stops moving around: it becomes ill. We are not designed to spend our lives lying on the couch. Our body is designed to stay active. *Born to run*, as Bruce Springsteen said.

Multiple Benefits

Some people, especially if they are in poor physical condition, believe that exercising is a sacrifice and that, rather than being good for you, it is a form of torture. People who think this way, and there are many, are only fooling themselves because the activity they perceive as damaging is actually beneficial to them.

In fact, the human body loves exercise. In the cardiovascular system, it raises the level of HDL (good cholesterol) and reduces the level of harmful triglycerides; it helps lower blood pressure; it helps fight overweight and obesity; it favors insulin activity and reduces the risk of developing diabetes. In short, it has an enormous impact on heart attack and stroke prevention, so much so that people who exercise regularly at the age of fifty can expect to live nearly four years longer than sedentary people. And these are only some of the benefits of exercise.

In the nervous system, it acts as an antidote to stress. It helps overcome depression, probably because it triggers the release of euphoria-producing endorphins in the brain. And it may reduce the risk of Alzheimer's by nearly 50 percent, according to a study by the Karolinska Institute that looked into the lifestyle and diseases of almost 1,500 men over thirty for five years. A 50 percent reduction means that for every ten potential cases of Alzheimer's, five may be avoided (or delayed long enough not to be detected in the study) and only five may occur.

As for cancer, it has been found that exercise reduces the risk of developing breast and colorectal tumors, two of the most common in the West. But we lack the data to determine whether it also prevents other forms of cancer.

We do know that it prevents osteoporosis, since many types of exercise strengthen muscles, which in turn strengthens bones and reduces the risk of fractures. We know it is good for balance and motor control, which is very important for the elderly to feel secure and to prevent falls and fractures. We know it improves intellectual performance. And, paradoxically, it is restful. That's right: exercise does not wear you out; it is restful. You might feel tired right after you exercise, but later on you are likely to feel more energetic. All of this has been confirmed by many studies.

But of all the benefits of exercise, certainly the most important one is that it encourages you to take responsibility for your own health. This is something we see, for example, in people who have suffered a heart attack. If you start exercising in the first few weeks, rather than give in, it's a sign that you are on the road to recovery, that your health will improve, and you will be able to lead a normal life, perhaps even better than before having the heart attack.

Exercise is not a quick fix like taking a pill; rather it requires the active participation of the patient. And anyone who is motivated to exercise will surely be motivated to control his weight, to quit smoking, to manage his cholesterol. If you care enough to exercise, your overall health is likely to be better. If you don't exercise, it is likely to be worse.

It's Not Hard to Get Started

It's not hard to get started. I have seen sixty-year-olds who had never exercised in their lives suddenly become aware of its importance—they start running and there is no stopping them. Quitting smoking, or drinking less, or eating better forces you to break habits that have become ingrained over years.

But exercise does not require a break with anything. You only need to be willing to start walking. And it has the great advantage, unlike quitting smoking or dieting, of immediate gratification because you start to feel better right away.

If you decide to start exercising, you are likely to have a few questions. What is the healthiest exercise that I can do? Is it true that there is nothing better than swimming or that a short walk every day is enough? Is a strenuous activity healthier than a more relaxed one? How many times a week should I exercise? Is more always better, or is there a point at which I no longer get any additional benefit from pushing myself?

These very questions have been raised by the researchers working on preventive health, and there have been dozens of studies aimed at coming up with answers to them based on sound scientific evidence. The findings show that there are three variables that affect the benefits of exercise: intensity (how hard you work out), frequency (how many times a week), and duration (how long per session).

The More Intense the Better?

We used to think exercise had to be intense to be healthy. But studies done on volunteers who get no exercise apart from walking—just walking—show that we were wrong: we now know that even moderate exercise can be a tremendous boon for your health. This does not mean that there are no differences between intense and moderate activity. What it means is that intensity is not everything, not even the most important thing.

What matters most is the duration and frequency of exercise, according to the findings from the studies. Thus, moderate intensity over a longer period of time is better for your health than a short burst of intense activity. Which is great news because the most common reason people quit exercising is that they find it too strenuous rather than too time-consuming. So, if their doctor recommends that they choose a lighter form of exercise, they may stick to it and in the end gain more from it. Still, all else being equal, the more vigorous the activity the more energy you burn, the more you crank up your cardiorespiratory system, and the greater the gains for your health.

We have several ways of measuring the intensity of exercise. In the stress tests we perform, we use METs, or metabolic equivalents: 1 MET equals the amount of oxygen—and thus calories—a person's body consumes while at rest. In adults, moderate exercise such as fast walking would be equivalent to 4 to 6 METs. Above 6 METs, we are talking about intense activity such as running. And the maximum oxygen consumption for a man of fifty is usually between 9 and 10 METs. METs are useful in laboratory conditions, but they have their limits. When you are out exercising on your own, you have no way of knowing how much oxygen you are consuming.

For real fitness fanatics who want to achieve what we call the target heart rate (THR), you can wear a pulsemeter, which constantly monitors your rate. I do not recommend pulsemeters for most people who exercise because they can lead to an obsession with your pulse. But for athletes who push their bodies to the limit, such as marathon runners or mountain climbers, it can be very useful. I wear a pulsemeter when I cycle up big mountain passes such as Tourmalet or Galibier in the Pyrenees or Alps during my summer holidays because I know my limit is 150 beats per minute and that if I exceed that, I won't make it to the top. But that is the only time I wear a pulsemeter when I exercise.

To find your target heart rate, you start by calculating what we call the maximum heart rate (MHR), which you get by subtracting your age from 220. For a forty-year-old, then, the MHR would be 180 beats per minute (220 minus 40). This rate is the maximum that you can reach in a sprint, for example. Target heart rate, which is sustainable during prolonged aerobic activity such as riding a bicycle over a mountain pass, lies between 60 percent and 75 percent of maximum frequency, as determined by the American Heart Association. Thus, a forty-year-old should be able to maintain a steady heart rate of between 108 (60 percent of 180) and 135 (75 percent). However, these numbers are only rough, and a fit person might not reach 108 whereas someone who is out of shape quickly hits 135 when doing the same exercise.

Objective measures of the intensity of exercise like MET and heart rate do not play a major role in preventing cardiovascular accidents. More important, as studies in the United States done at Harvard University and Duke University have shown, is the subjective perception you have from exercising. In other words, if you are not used to exercising and you feel worn-out after a 2-kilometer walk, you have gained nearly as much from the standpoint of prevention as an athlete who runs, say, a half marathon. This is great news because it means that someone who tires quickly needn't feel daunted by the thought of exercise; they still stand to gain a lot from a workout without performing superhuman feats.

How Often and For How Long?

More important than the intensity of the exercise is the duration and frequency with which you do it. A typical example is someone who works out on the weight machine at the gym, puts 20 kilograms on each arm to build up the biceps to the max, and then promptly maxes out after 10 curls. This same person, if they put just 5 pounds on each arm, and then maxes after 20 curls, would strengthen their muscles too. Though it might feel like you are barely lifting any weight at all, the number of curls is much more important than the weight you lift.

Twenty minutes of vigorous exercise three times a week has been shown to have a significant positive impact on cardiovascular health. Thirty minutes four times a week is even better. This is actually the basic recommendation of the American Heart Association, the American College of Sports Medicine, and the U.S. Centers for Disease Control: thirty minutes of moderate exercise at least four times a week. If you find thirty minutes too little and want to make it an hour, that is just as good or better, especially for your blood cholesterol levels. And the same applies if instead of four days a week you prefer to exercise every day.

You needn't get these thirty to sixty minutes in one go, but rather they can be spread throughout the day because in the end what counts is the total minutes of exercise. And you can count as exercise the time you spend cleaning house, gardening, washing the car, walking to the subway—as long as you walk fast—or climbing the stairs instead of taking the elevator up to the office.

We do not know if you get any additional health benefits beyond one hour of daily exercise. Clearly, there must be a point of peak benefit after which health no longer improves no matter how hard you work out. We lack conclusive studies to know if this peak is one hour a day, more than an hour, or even less. But from my personal experience, having done a lot of sports for many years, especially tennis and cycling, I would say that beyond an hour a day the benefits are mainly psychological: you feel very fit and full of energy.

There is no need to do the same kind of exercise every day. For many people, it is easier to integrate exercise into their schedule, more pleasant, too, alternating a number of activities, like going to the pool two days, taking a thirty-minute walk another, and going Rollerblading, hiking, or skiing on the weekend.

I have seen patients with tight schedules who prefer two one-hour sessions a week to four half-hour sessions, in the belief that the effect is the same. Or they do nothing from Monday to Friday and leave it all for Saturday and Sunday. Of course, this is better than nothing. But it seems that it is not as beneficial as doing less exercise more frequently. The reason is that the effects of exercise are similar to those of a drug: it acts on cholesterol, insulin, blood pressure. In fact, if we had a drug with the same effects as exercise, and so few side effects, we would prescribe it for everyone in the world. But we would prescribe one pill a day, and no less often than every two days, to maintain constant action on cholesterol, insulin, and tension throughout the week. Leaving all your exercise for the weekend would be like taking such pills, even in a double dose, Saturday and Sunday only. You might get a big boost on Monday or Tuesday, but from Wednesday on the effects will start to wane.

What Exercise Is Best for Me?

I often deal with patients who tell me, "I know I should take up some sport, but I don't know what sport to do." Before you decide, you should know that there are two types of exercises, aerobic and anaerobic. Although both have salutary effects, the effects are different.

Aerobic exercises raise the demand for oxygen from your muscles. You know you are doing aerobic exercise when you need to breathe faster and deeper. This is because your heart rate accelerates to supply your muscles with extra oxygen. Since the temperature of muscles rises for the same reason any machine gets hot because it is burning energy, soon the body starts to sweat in order to get rid of excess heat. Aerobic exercises are ideal for improving cardiorespiratory health, building endurance, and burning off calories. Examples include walking, running, swimming, skating, cycling, and, as the name suggests, aerobics.

On the other hand, you know you are doing anaerobic exercise when you feel your muscles straining, often to the point of trembling or hurting, in order to overcome some form of resistance. Anaerobic exercises are ideal for strengthening muscles and bones, and are especially beneficial for older persons insofar as they help prevent osteoporosis and falling. Plus, they increase glucose consumption by your muscles, which is good for people with diabetes. But anaerobic exercises can cause a sharp increase in blood pressure, so people with hypertension should approach them with caution and consult their doctor first. Examples of anaerobic exercises include weight lifting, push-ups or sit-ups, as well as specific aspects of aerobic activities such as climbing a hill on a bicycle.

Aerobic and anaerobic activities are complementary and, except in cases of contraindication, as in hypertensive people who do not have their blood pressure under tight control, the ideal thing is to combine the two to obtain the greatest benefits for your health.

But when someone who has not done any exercise for years asks me for advice on which sport to do, as a rule I suggest they start by walking. It's the perfect activity for starting to get fit because almost everyone can do it: it is as easy as getting off the bus one or two stops early or parking your car at the far end of the lot; the risk of injury is minimal, it requires no special equipment except a pair of comfortable shoes, and it's free. The only thing you must remember is that walking with the aim of getting exercise is not the same as going for a stroll. You must do it long enough and fast enough to stimulate your cardiorespiratory system. You can listen to music through headphones to liven up your walk if you like, but it's no good stopping to look in shop windows or admire the scenery. If you do not feel like you are making an effort, even after covering the distance you set out to do, you are only making half the distance in cardiovascular protection.

Thus I often tell my patients: "You walk two miles a day, a distance that someone in shape can do in half an hour at a fast pace. Time yourself and then each month try to cut a minute off your time. When you reach the point where you really feel you're getting tired, you have reached the ideal speed for your cardiovascular health."

Do I Need to See the Doctor Before I Start?

For some people, of course, walking sounds somehow not challenging enough. Once they get the idea in their head that after years of sedentary life they are going to start exercising, they go for broke. Which can be a dangerous proposition: in the United States it is estimated that between 1 and 3 percent of heart attacks victims are engaged, at the time of the attack, in strenuous exercise they are not prepared for. That does not mean that exercise is inadvisable, not even for such people. All it means is that you cannot start off in overdrive without being aware of your limitations, just as you cannot learn to climb starting with Mont Blanc. So for some people contemplating certain activities, it is advisable to consult a doctor first.

As a general rule, anyone who has previously led a sedentary life should start with an activity of moderate intensity before tackling anything more strenuous. Men under forty-five and women under fifty-five who do not smoke or have any other known cardiovascular risk factors, such as high cholesterol or hypertension, can begin without consulting a doctor. The age difference between men and women is due to the fact that heart attack becomes a real risk factor about ten years later in females than in males (although we don't know if the reason is the protective effects of estrogen until menopause in women or the aggressive effects of androgens like testosterone in men, or both).

From the age of forty-five for men and fifty-five for women, or younger in the case of those with known cardiovascular risk factors, it is advisable to visit the family doctor to ensure your exercise program is safe for you. In special cases, such as people who have been diagnosed with a cardiovascular condition or have a family history of heart failure, it is advisable to see the cardiologist directly, who may want to do a stress test to determine whether your heart can withstand exercise without risk.

But if you take these basic precautions, anyone can do themselves a huge favor by getting the sorts of exercise you got as a child on the playground: running, jumping, and shouting, and following the basic instincts of the human species.

CHAPTER SIXTEEN

Exercise, Part 2

. . . AND HOW TO KEEP GOING

I have yet to encounter a single patient who disputed the idea that exercise would be good for their health. Not one. But I've heard all kinds of arguments, and also reasonable doubts, from patients who say they accept the benefits of physical activity as an abstract idea, but they have tight schedules, other priorities, and they don't see how that abstract idea can apply to them. They'd like to be able to say, yeah, I will exercise, but they can't. They think they can't.

What can a doctor do in these cases? The first thing is to remember that we are at the service of the patient, not the God of Physical Activity, so we must respect the freedom of each patient to do what they deem best for themselves and not try to impose four workouts a week against their will. But I think we should inform them of the benefits of exercise and the risks of being sedentary and answer any questions they may have regarding what sort of workout is best for them and how to make it part of their daily lives. And having gone through all that, I often find people who had said that physical activity was not for them and then leave my office with the will at least to give it a shot. When they come back to see me a few months later, some are active and feel better and some have even become genuine converts, having gone from barely walking to and from the car to not being able to live without their daily dose of exercise.

The Imperfect Excuse: "I Don't Have Time"

For many patients, the immediate reaction when you tell them that they would benefit from getting some exercise is to say they don't have the time. They might think that's so, but it never is. We already talked about this in chapter 4, but it's so important that we are going to say it again: everyone finds the time to do what they really want to do. So if you want to exercise and take care of your health you will find time to do so; if you cannot, it is because you do not want to—because you do not have the motivation. You have the time—it's just that you spend it doing other things.

In my personal experience, exercise does not take time away from other activities. Quite the contrary: it makes the time devoted to other activities more productive. Many patients have told me as much: after starting to exercise regularly, they feel better physically and sharper intellectually; they have more energy and can concentrate better.

Physical activity comes in so many forms that anyone can find a hole in their schedule for it. You can exercise almost anytime, almost anywhere. I have patients who opt for an exercise bike at home because they find it easier to combine physical activity and family life. Others get up early in the morning to go running or swimming. I have another who signed up for the gym three days a week at midday, but since he often has business lunches, he settled on two days at the gym and another workout on the weekend. I do not mean that any of these solutions is right for you: these are only examples to show that anyone can find a way.

Your work schedule permitting, before lunch is a perfect time for a bit of exercise. But if you can get away from the job at noon, and rather than an hour- or an hour-and-a-half lunch, exercise for half an hour and eat in half an hour, you'll come out ahead in both personal and work terms: you burn more calories and eat less; your mood improves; you perform better on the job. A pre-lunch workout also has the advantage of inhibiting substances in the brain that stimulate appetite, so it helps you to eat less and avoid putting on weight. After lunch your blood goes to your digestive system, so it is not such a good time for your muscles to be demanding extra oxygen.

Moreover, scheduling your workout usually at the same time of day helps you to be consistent and stick with it. People who exercise whenever they find a moment, without fixing the day and time, are more likely to give it up.

"I'm Too Old"

When I deal with elderly patients, they often say they are not up to exercise anymore. A seventy-five-year-old naturally has neither the energy nor the flexibility of a twenty-five-year-old. They may have some chronic condition such as arthritis or back pain and be afraid that exercise will make the pain even worse. They may have problems with their balance. But even if they can no longer do somersaults like their grandchildren or exercise with the same intensity as they once did, exercise is as healthy for the elderly as it is for younger people. Perhaps even more so. It is well proven that even light physical activity improves cardiorespiratory capacity and slows intellectual decline among elderly people. For patients who suffer chronic pain, remaining inactive does not relieve pain and may even aggravate it. For people with mobility problems in their legs, for example, due to knee pain, there are exercises for the trunk and arms. If you have problems with your balance, stay away from the treadmill, which is easy to fall off, and work out on the exercise bike. And if the mere idea of exercise seems over-whelming, you should remember that there is no need to wear yourself out. To get started, it's enough to take a short walk, and any progress, no matter how little, is a step in the right direction. If you live on the fifth floor, for example, try climbing the stairs, and if you run out of steam on the third, take the elevator up the rest of the way. That's better than nothing. Often the main obstacle elderly people face when it comes to exercise is not physical but mental. In other words, it is not that they cannot do it physically but that they think: I can't, I'm too old, my back hurts too much. In fact, this mental block to physical effort occurs not only in older people but among people of all ages.

I have experienced it myself cycling up mountains in the Pyrenees and Alps. In 2005, at the age of sixty-two, I climbed Mortirolo in Italy, with 15 percent gradients and reckoned by cyclists to be the toughest climb in Europe. The previous year, I did Stelvio, also in Italy, a 23-kilometer climb to an altitude of 2,758 meters (9,050 feet) above sea level, where you can feel the oxygen start to thin. And in 2003 I did Télégraphe and Galibier in the French Alps in one day. Ten years earlier I would not have been able to do any of these climbs because I did not feel up to it. In fact, Mont Ventoux in France, in 1990 when I was forty-seven, was the hardest climb I ever did, and not because it is so steep or so high but because I was not mentally prepared. However, I did it again in 2007 without any difficulties, this time with my daughter!

So I have come to the conclusion that when it comes to physical challenges, we accord age more importance than it deserves and we forget that far more important than age is the confidence you have in your own potential.

In short, whether an eighty-five-year-old with arthritis exercises or not depends less on their age or their condition than on their confidence in their own ability to do it.

"But Isn't That Dangerous?"

I remember one very hot summer day I was training for the Tourmalet climb on the hill up to the castle above Cardona, a town in Catalonia where I usually spend my vacations. It was almost noon, when a beer truck pulled alongside and slowed down.

"But, *hombre*, are you out of your mind, out here on a bike with this sun?" the driver smirked.

"I'm training."

"Training? Be smart, *hombre*—go home and have a nice cold beer. Don't you see what you're doing is bad for you? And riding up this hill. You'll get a heart attack!"

"Hey, I'm a doctor," I finally told him. "I know what I'm doing."

"So you're a doctor? Well, you know what? If I ever get sick, you can be sure you won't see me in your office." Then he drove off and that was the last I saw of him.

That's just an anecdote, but it illustrates a widespread view that exercise can be counterproductive. Actually, the beer distributor was right that when you exercise you put a strain on your whole cardiorespiratory system. You breathe harder, your heart beats faster, and your maximum blood pressure can rise between 20 and 50 millimeters of mercury. In stress tests with patients at my office, we have seen highs of 180, a level which is no cause for concern when we are talking about strenuous activity. Worrisome would be a constant 180 with peaks up to 220, for instance. But we do not believe a high of 180 for a few minutes has any significant adverse effects. On the contrary, by exerting the cardiorespiratory system, you lower the level at which your maximum blood pressure stabilizes for the rest of the day—specifically, the maximum drops by 5 to 10 millimeters of mercury with regular exercise—and thus you reduce the risk of cardiovascular accident. Good cholesterol rises by about 5 percent, while bad cholesterol falls by about 5 percent, and the risk of developing diabetes drops significantly. And people who have already survived one heart attack, who are often afraid of exerting themselves, with regular exercise, may reduce their risk of another heart attack; in other words, recent data suggests that exercise may prevent 1 in 5 reinfarctions. So we have a whole range of figures showing that the benefits far outweigh the risks.

But it is true: if you are not careful, exercise can entail risk. That's why it's so important for people who lead sedentary lives to consult their doctor before embarking on a program of strenuous exercise and, if necessary, to take a stress test. By following these rules of thumb, and taking things gradually, anyone can exercise within their own limits without fear of cardiovascular accident.

"What If I Injure Myself?"

In fact, the most common problem associated with exercise is musculoskeletal injuries, for example, affecting your muscles, bones, tendons (which connect muscles to bones), or ligaments (ties between the bones in your joints). Such injuries may seem minor compared with cardiovascular accidents, but they can be very serious. About 50 percent of people who exercise regularly suffer a major injury at some point. And some of those will be left with some permanent damage, most commonly to their knees, feet, or back.

We often shrug off injuries as inevitable. Typically, we tell ourselves things like: "So I put my foot down wrong and got a sprained ankle"; or "My knee? Oh, I just slipped and pulled the ligaments"; or "I just didn't see the other skier, so now I have a broken fibula." But the truth is, the vast majority of injuries are preventable—if you follow a few common sense rules.

The first rule is, after a prolonged period of inactivity, start easy and gradually ratchet up the effort. People typically want to go at full throttle as soon as they decide to start exercising, a tendency I have seen in many patients. They don't care if they haven't moved a muscle in ten years. The attitude is: Ready, Set, Go: six miles the first day! I always tell such people that they can do strenuous exercise but not the first day; it's better to start slowly.

Many injuries happen precisely because people try to do more than their body is ready for. You overestimate your abilities, set unrealistic goals, ignore the signs of fatigue and pain in your own body. These are distress signals from your muscles, tendons, or joints, and if you don't heed their call, you'll end up back on the couch—only this time with a bandage, an analgesic, an anti-inflammatory, and pain that, before you got off the couch in the first place, you never had. So if you feel pain, especially if you have an injury, rather than pushing your body, it's better to stop; you can resume exercising when your body is ready a few days later. An injury is always a risk when ignored.

"Oh, it's nothing, just a nuisance, but it doesn't stop me from doing anything," someone might say and forget that that muscle or joint needs time to recover, and an injury that starts out being minor, if not given proper repose, can grow into a chronic injury.

In the end, minor injuries which, due to ignorance or negligence, become major injuries are one of the prime reasons people quit doing sports: Sunday soccer players forced to give up the game due to bad knees or ankles, tennis players with chronic elbow or shoulder pain, runners whose knees give out. . .

So if you get an injury, however slight, it is best to take a break. And if rest doesn't cure it, see your doctor. If the recovery is long, look for some alternative activity that does not overstress the damaged muscle or joint. While running might seem an innocuous activity, it causes about 75 percent of sports injuries, so it is crucial for runners to wear the right shoes to absorb the impact of each step and avoid putting too much stress on your ankles and knees. It is also highly advisable to spend a few minutes stretching before and after any vigorous activity. And to minimize the risk of injury, you should exercise often: it has been shown that people who exercise sporadically are more prone to injury than regular exercisers.

Apart from watching out for injuries, you should also be aware of the risk of exercise becoming an obsession. This is a very common problem but may become as serious as an addiction. I have seen people who have made working out the center of their lives, sacrificing their careers and personal life to keep up with an intense exercise program, happily turning their backs on friendships; I even know one such case that ended up in divorce. So, exercise is extremely healthy—it is just about the best thing you can do for health—but it entails risks of injury and social isolation that one should be aware of in order to avoid them.

"I Don't Like Physical Activity"

I often have patients who say, "I know I should exercise, but I simply don't like it." Some try swimming and give up because it is boring; others try running but get discouraged because it is tiring; others cannot motivate themselves to try anything at all. Such people often assume that their sedentary lifestyle is part of their nature.

Still, in my experience as a doctor, nearly everyone ends up finding some kind of physical activity they enjoy. People that once considered themselves incurable couch potatoes may even go from one extreme to another and end up being exercise nuts. But it is true that there are some people, a minority, in my opinion, who simply do not like to exercise.

Such cases are complicated because when physical activity is not rewarding, you are not likely to stick with it for long. You try it, you stop, and you do not try again until the following year when you go back to the doctor and she reminds you again of all the benefits of a physically active life and the dangers of a sedentary one. So what we need to ask ourselves is how we can make exercise gratifying for these people.

One option is to recommend something easy, like walking, so that they do not get discouraged, and the simple fact of feeling how their health improves may prove rewarding enough. But some people still find a half-hour walk a day a real drag, and they dislike wearing headphones, so listening to the radio or music is not an option as a means of warding off boredom.

Something that has worked for many of my patients is to get an exercise bike for home, so they can get their workout while watching TV. Another good way to fight tedium is to go to the gym or pool or for a walk, at least once a week, with a friend or family member. Exercising with someone else can be a lot more fun than doing it alone.

Another effective strategy is to vary the type of physical activity that you do. Going out for a run or a walk four days a week can become boring, so many people prefer to walk two days and go swimming or cycling, for example, the other two days. A change of activity also has the advantage of exercising different muscle groups and reducing the risk of injury from repetitive action.

Is Swimming the Best Exercise?

Among all the recommended forms of exercise, swimming is probably one of the best. It is wonderful for improving cardiorespiratory capacity, especially when you do the crawl. It is wonderful for strengthening muscles and thus your bones. It helps relieve the pain and stiffness of arthritis and lower back pain. The risk of injury is minimal. And it's great for staying active while recovering from an injury from another activity.

Yet, despite all these benefits, it is a mistake to swim just because you think you should when you have a choice of other types of exercise that you enjoy more. Experience shows that most people who take up a physical activity they do not enjoy end up losing interest and eventually quitting. So if you do not like swimming, you should look for an alternative.

Walking is a great way to get fit for people just starting to exercise. It is also good for people who are already in shape, but you must always remember to keep up your pace in order to get the maximum cardiorespiratory benefits.

Running works your cardiorespiratory system harder, but the risk of long-term injury is also greater because of the impact on your joints each time your foot hits the ground. This is especially true when you run on hard surfaces such as asphalt or cement. To reduce the risk, doctors recommend proper shoes to absorb the impact, as well as running on softer surfaces such as dirt roads, a beach, or a running track.

Cycling is also a good option, although, as with walking, you need to remind yourself to keep up your pace: if you do not ride hard and long enough, your heart will not be getting the intended benefits.

The American Heart Association also recommends Rollerblading and ice skating as aerobic exercises that are as healthy as cycling or running. Skating has the advantages of being fun; it burns a huge amount of calories; it reduces stress; and it is great for strengthening buttocks and thigh muscles.

Team sports such as soccer or basketball, on the other hand, are less advisable as a means of getting regular exercise. The reason is simply practical: while a game a week in the park makes for a great complement to your regular exercise program, it is not easy to get all the people you need to make up two teams together four times a week.

What Goals Do I Set for Myself?

Two of the most common mistakes people make when they start exercising is to set goals that are too high and to try to reach their goals too quickly. Some people do not seem to realize that at fifty they cannot do the same things they did at twenty. You might have been a track star in college, but you would be foolish to try to show your friends how high you used to jump without getting yourself back in shape first. Likewise, you are asking for trouble if you take exercise as a competition starting the first day of your second youth. People who do so are prime candidates for injury, frustration, and failure.

To avoid these mistakes, it is worth remembering that the goal is not to win an Olympic medal or to be the champion of anything but something far more important: to improve your health. And that is not something that can be achieved in 10 seconds, like winning a 100-meter sprint; it's more like a long-distance race in which goals are reached in the longer term. Bearing this in mind, anyone can, if they like, set themselves specific goals, so long as they are within reason. But these goals will vary widely, depending on the person and the type of exercise they do.

Your particular aim might be simply to work out four times every week; or it could be to run a thousand meters in under 3 minutes 30 seconds. In my case, it is to bike up a major pass in the Pyrenees or the Alps every summer, a goal that keeps me motivated to work out the rest of the year.

"Won't I Get Fat If I Quit Working Out?"

If you follow these basic recommendations—find a form of exercise that is rewarding for you, fit it into a schedule compatible with work and family life, set reasonable goals, do not neglect injuries—the risk of quitting and returning to a life of inactivity is low. There are more people that start smoking again or have a hard time sticking to a diet than people who quit exercising once they start. Even so, I have patients that fear the musculature they build up with exercise will go soft and turn to fat as soon as they stop being so active. They may be thinking of Marlon Brando, such a hunk when he was young and so obese when he was old. But their fears are unfounded.

Muscles and fat are two distinct types of tissue and one cannot transform into another. Your muscles will never turn to fat any more than your fat will ever turn to muscle; so if you lose your muscles, you will not necessarily gain a paunch. It is true that muscles can atrophy when no longer exercised and that if you exercise less and do not reduce your calorie intake, you will eventually get fatter. But that is not the worst thing about giving up exercise.

The worst thing is that all the health risks you were keeping at bay come home to roost: bad cholesterol rises again; blood pressure goes back up; you lose agility; you have less energy; the risk of diabetes shoots up. And all those benefits that you fought so hard to achieve—and that you will have to fight to regain in the future—start to fade away in a few weeks.

CHAPTER SEVENTEEN

Stress

LIVING ON THE EDGE

I have never in my life seen a patient who has had a heart attack or some other cardiovascular incident that was due to stress alone. There is always some other cause to explain the condition. It could be high cholesterol, or diabetes, or smoking, or hypertension. Any of these risk factors can be sufficient to cause a cardiovascular accident. But not stress. If you suffer from stress and nothing else, you will not have a heart attack.

However, though stress does not cause heart attacks, it can trigger them. So a person who has other significant risk factors in addition to being subject to acute stress is in the danger zone.

There are countless cases of people whose condition is basically stable until a change in their situation tips them over the edge. For example, the person who dies of a heart attack a few days after the death of their spouse and we will hear people say "they were such a close couple," when the heart attack was brought on not by love but by stress. Or the defendant who keels over during cross-examination in court. Or the woman who ended up in the hospital the night of her sixty-fifth birthday because her friends had prepared a surprise party, and when she got home and switched on the light, suddenly she found a dozen people shouting congratulations and got the fright of her life.

The idea of being frightened to death refers precisely to this: a moment of sudden stress that, for a vulnerable person, can cause a heart attack.

Strong Emotions

But the stress response, despite its bad reputation, is not an unhealthy reaction; nor is it always negative. In fact, it is a natural function not just of humans but of animals in general, in which the organism responds with a massive release of hormones such as adrenaline and cortisol to a fight or flight situation, to help us escape or confront a danger.

So we should be thankful for stress because if this survival mechanism had failed just once in one of our ancestors in the last 500 million years, we might not have the good fortune to be here today.

Moreover, a certain level of stress can be pleasurable, as anyone who has ever enjoyed a roller-coaster ride or a horror film will testify. Many of us find that an element of tension makes us feel more alive, boosting our energy level and our desire to do things. There are even extreme cases of people for whom the excitement of the stress response is so important that they choose to lead a high-adrenaline life as skydivers, war correspondents, or Formula One drivers. And though there are plenty of people who would gladly avoid strong emotions, stress is such a natural biological reaction that there is really no possibility of living without it. Even happy experiences are likely to involve stress: getting married is stressful, and so is going on holiday, shopping for Christmas presents or preparing a dinner for fifteen guests, not to mention rearing children, moving to a new house, making it to the end of the month, or being stuck in a traffic jam 100 miles from home on a Sunday afternoon.

So the problem we have with stress is not about eradicating it from our lives but about learning to control it so that a necessary natural response does not become a harmful reaction.

Acute Stress, Chronic Stress

The first thing to be clear about, in controlling stress, is that there are different types of harmful stress that have different origins and different effects on our health. On the one hand, there are episodes of acute stress: for example, when someone loses his temper to such an extent that he starts acting irrationally. A situation like this is rather like a short circuit in the brain; it is as if the neurons that control our rational responses had lost contact with the neurons that control our emotional responses, and the result is an outburst of primary emotional behavior without any rational restraint. During such episodes—which are usually brief, lasting only seconds or minutes—the levels of adrenaline and cortisol in the blood go shooting up. In people with weakened heart and arteries, these episodes can be fatal.

I remember the case of a patient who was so annoyed with his boss one day that he climbed onto a desk where everyone could see him and started denouncing the boss's failings so everyone could hear him. But what they all heard was his voice suddenly dry up and what they saw a second later was him keel over and fall off the desk. The cause was adrenaline.

Adrenaline has a powerful coagulant effect and can trigger a heart attack in the same way that smoking can; it also interferes with the heart rate and can produce a fatal arrhythmia. However, for people who are in good cardiovascular shape, sporadic surges of adrenaline do not seem to have any significant adverse effects on health, though they may have on their personal relationships.

Then there is a second type of stress, occasioned by a traumatic event such as a divorce or the death of a loved one, which often extends over days or weeks and is also accompanied by increased adrenaline secretion. Though the stress hormones do not usually go up as much as in a sudden fit of rage, they can still bring on a heart attack in someone whose cardiovascular health is poor, as it often does in older people who have recently been widowed.

But there is yet another kind of stress, and this is the one that has the most serious impact on health: persistent stress does not ease off in a few minutes or a few weeks but tends to become chronic. With persistent stress there is no surge in adrenaline secretion; instead, the person is living at the very limit of what they can endure, in a permanent state of dissatisfaction, either because of problems at work or at home, in the family, or because they feel lonely, or all of these together. And it is not uncommon for it all to end in a heart attack.

It is not clear whether this type of chronic stress can directly cause a cardiovascular accident, as the levels of adrenaline and cortisol levels are not as high as in acute stress. But there is evidence that it makes people eat more and, worse still, smoke more, drink more, let themselves go—and when we add up all the consequences of chronic stress, the impact on health is enormous. Mood and psychological balance are so important for the evolution of a heart condition that one of the first questions I always ask my patients is if they feel depressed or stressed, and about 60 percent of them tell me that they live with stress. And half of those say they live with unbearable stress.

Of course, these figures do not have the validity of a scientific study; they merely reflect what I see in my day-to-day work. But I feel sure that if we went out into the street and put the same question to 100 people chosen at random, we would not find 60 with chronic stress or 30 who are under unbearable stress. In other words, this form of stress may not directly trigger a heart attack, but it predisposes one to risk. It is, for many patients, the cause of the causes of a heart attack. And if we could eradicate chronic stress, no doubt we would drastically reduce the number of cardiovascular accidents.

Slaves to the Clock

Despite their differences, the different types of harmful stress have something in common: in all of them, the person loses control of what he or she does. This is what characterizes stress: instead of being free to decide what we want to do, the environment decides for us. The environment dominates us. At the root of most cases of chronic stress are too little time and too much ambition. If you do not have time to do everything you want to, and you want to do more than you can, you inevitably feel overwhelmed. And because time is limited—and this is part of the equation that we cannot change—limitless ambitions can only lead to a sense of frustration and a personal crisis.

I see a lot of people who start feeling stressed because of lack of time almost as soon as they get out of bed. It's eight a.m., they've just left home, they're stuck in traffic as usual, and they start fretting because they're going to get to work late. This kind of stress need not affect the health of a healthy person, though it certainly affects their quality of life. But some people live totally stressed lives, always right on the edge, doing everything at the last minute. And they probably need to stop for a moment and think why they are always in a hurry and how they can remedy that: perhaps by leaving home 10 minutes earlier, or accepting that they will arrive 10 minutes late, or perhaps thinking about what it is they really want to do.

Personally, no project I have ever done in a hurry has turned out well. Not one. Undue haste leads to mediocre results; the work may get finished on schedule, but from the standpoint of personal development, you have not achieved anything.

Recognizing Chronic Stress

The trouble is that chronic stress, if it is not nipped in the bud, is a monster that feeds itself: stress creates more stress. It is likely, for example, that if we are unable to manage our time, we will feel overwhelmed and stressed, causing us to sleep badly and wake up tired, making us feel even more overwhelmed and even more stressed. And if we start drinking endless cups of coffee to fight off drowsiness and keep up the pace—a very common reaction—we end up sleeping even worse, needing ever larger doses of caffeine and feeling even more overwhelmed.

As soon as stress becomes part of this vicious cycle, it is easy for the dynamic to intensify to the point where the threat of a threat is enough to make us feel overwhelmed: we no longer need to experience a stressful situation—the very idea is enough to make us panic. In some cases, the stress dynamic feeds back to such an extent that it gets totally out of control and ends up as the psychological equivalent of nuclear meltdown. And it can happen to anyone. There is no typical profile of the stress-vulnerable person. It affects men and women equally: Wall Street executives and factory workers—and also those of us who believe we are able to withstand any amount of pressure, who have never lost control and think we are immune to stress. Some people tend not to externalize their emotions, until one day they reach their limit and explode like a pressure cooker. And then, when they do, their colleagues turn around, amazed, and say, "Who would have imagined it? He always seemed so coolheaded."

The problem in modern urban societies is that though we interact with hundreds of people every day, many of us live alone, we have no one who will really listen to us, and in turn we probably do not listen to anyone, do not trust anyone, pursuing our own ambitions to the highest summit and heading unknowingly toward the abyss. And we fail to appreciate the impact of stress on our lives until the day we find we have a major health problem because no one has told us that the life we are leading is absurd, doing so much and enjoying so little. Or perhaps someone did try to tell us, but we didn't listen.

So I think it is important for everyone to have someone close to them, someone they trust and confide in, someone they listen to who can warn them and help them if they seem to be on a collision course. Because no one sees themselves impartially, and what usually happens with chronic stress is that we accept it as part of our life, and we think we are capable of putting up with it, until one day it crushes us.

There are various signs or symptoms that can help us identify incipient chronic stress, though none is unequivocal because they may reflect situations that have nothing to do with stress. The most obvious are physical symptoms like nail biting, clenching one's teeth, fatigue, headaches, digestive problems, and insomnia. The psychological symptoms, which tend to be more difficult to pinpoint but are no less important, include moodiness, anxiety, feeling pessimistic, feeling misunderstood or undervalued, sudden fits of tears or of laughter, and a desire to break with everything. When these symptoms are present with no obvious explanation for them, it is worth considering whether they may be due to stress, in order to try to deal with the situation before it enters into the dynamic of chronic stress. Recognizing the situation and deciding to do something about it is the most difficult part.

Most cases get out of control because people do not realize that their symptoms are due to stress or because they fail to see the implications and prefer to carry on as before. Once the stress situation has been identified as what it is, the most difficult step has been taken, and the next step is how to deal with it. More precisely, what people suffering from stress tend to ask is how to go about resolving it without having to change their job or their family.

Solutions That Do Not Work

Let's start with how not to go about it. The most common reaction to stress, the path millions of people take, is to self-medicate with alcohol. They come home at night and relax with a drink or two. And they do relax because alcohol is not a stimulant like coffee—it has the opposite effect: it depresses the nervous system. I am not against having a drink once in a while for pleasure. But to get into the habit of drinking every night in order to relax is a mistake. Because alcohol does not solve the problems that cause stress: it does not resolve your conflicts at work or at home, or your expecting to do too much in too little time, but only your excess tensions at the end of the day. At best it is a stopgap, and one that can actually interfere with your capacity to solve problems and aggravate the negative feelings associated with stress.

So alcohol is oblivion today, more worries tomorrow. Another non-solution, another very common mistake, is to get into the habit of taking tranquilizers. Tranquilizers have the same effect and the same drawbacks as alcohol: they may relax you, but they will not solve anything. And they are just as addictive. The mistake is to think that the pressure we all face in our daily lives is a disease that can be medicated away, when in fact it is a reality we have to learn to live with.

Other common reactions, which also fail to address the underlying problem, are to go outside for a cigarette or stop to eat a candy bar as a break from a stressful activity. Though these things can provide temporary relief, even prevent a crisis of acute stress, they cannot break the cycle of stress because chronic stress is not a storm that builds up and rains itself out in fifteen minutes but a whole high-pressure system that takes much longer to evolve and much longer to resolve.

Solutions That *Do* Work

For patients who come to me suffering from stress, I usually recommend three steps: relaxation techniques, exercise, and meditation. In fact, I often advise them to take up yoga, which is in some ways a synthesis of all three. In my hospital we have even opened a unit that offers yoga as a therapy for stressed patients. Some are surprised at first: "Yoga? Me? Really, doctor, it would never have occurred to me." But most are so discontented with their lives that they accept the idea. And the results are spectacular.

With yoga they regain physical control over their bodies, improving their flexibility and sense of balance, and, above all, control of their minds because they learn to relax by means of deep breathing techniques and disconnect from the hustle and bustle. Yoga is a way of helping them take control of their lives, enabling them to decide what they want to do with their time instead of letting the environment decide for them.

And even if people choose not to sign up for yoga, relaxation techniques based on control of breathing are always worthwhile. They are not difficult to learn and are useful both for avoiding acute stress and for preventing or overcoming chronic stress. An additional advantage is that they can be used discreetly in a whole range of situations, from a tense business meeting to a long line at the supermarket or a crush on the subway.

Basically, it is a question of learning to breathe slowly and deeply, moving your diaphragm, the muscle that separates your chest from your abdomen, rather than moving your shoulders, so that it is not your rib cage but your abdomen that goes in and out.

In cases where lack of sleep is one of the links in the stress cycle, it is also worth trying to recover a good sleep pattern. But it is a mistake to attach too much importance to sleep. A common mistake, of course: some people become obsessed with their difficulty in sleeping, and the obsession ends up being worse than the insomnia. I am not saying that a good night's sleep is not important, but there are plenty of cases of sleep disorders that are not associated with stress. And, in fact, the opposite of being stressed is not resting but relaxing. So rest is not a universal cure for stress. It is really only useful when the stress is accompanied by physical exhaustion.

Another thing that has proved very useful is physical exercise, especially as a preventive measure with people who are not yet caught up in the cycle of chronic stress; we have found that exercising several times a week helps get rid of tension and provides a kind of immunity from psychological stress. Of course, some people prefer gentler techniques such as meditation. Any of these options is valid if the result is that you feel relaxed, and each of us can choose the one that works best for us, according to our temperament, physical condition, and mood.

Time to Think

A final piece of advice I like to give to people suffering from stress is that they set aside some time every day, half an hour, for example, just for themselves, to think. Simply to think. It may sound strange as a medical treatment because thought is not something that can be prescribed like a pill or implanted in an operating theater like a pacemaker; it doesn't even need a teacher, as yoga does, and it's cheaper than a Band-Aid, but the therapeutic results are astounding.

Every year I see a whole host of patients who have let themselves be pushed along by the pressures of the world around them until they are literally sick at heart. They eat badly, they smoke, they are stressed, they punish their bodies, and usually they do not even know why they do it. These are people who have achieved outstanding success at the professional level but have completely lost control of their lives. But the ones who, after a heart attack, start to think about what they are doing, to ask themselves whether it makes sense for them, often manage to regain control of their lives, and this has a far greater impact on their health and well-being than any drug can have.

In fact, devoting a little time each day to thinking is something I would recommend to everyone: advice that I myself—and I do not consider myself an especially stressed person—

follow. I make a point of getting up early so as to have some time for myself first thing in the morning because I have the impression that in the world today there is too much haste and not enough reflection.

It is hardly surprising that chronic stress is such a prevalent modern disease because we live in a tremendously fast-paced world that leaves us next to no time to think about where we are, or where we are going, or what our goals are, or how to attain them. The world is changing so fast that the speed at which change occurs often outstrips our ability to adapt. So the best thing we can do is lift our foot off the accelerator, live in less of a headlong rush, and reclaim the capacity to decide what we want to do with our time.

CHAPTER EIGHTEEN

Emotions

HAPPINESS AS LIFE INSURANCE

I have always been skeptical of theories that claim that the mind controls the body, that the body in turn controls the mind, that the origin of many organic diseases is psychological imbalance, and that what we ought to be treating are not the symptoms of the illness but the underlying psychological imbalance. I still think that most of these theories have no scientific basis and are actually dangerous because they lead some people to spend their money on esoteric therapies that simply do not work when there are other treatments that are known to be effective which would do them far more good.

At the moment, though, I have a patient with metastatic cancer who has a tremendous desire to live. When he was first diagnosed with cancer, the prognosis was very bad. Now, three years later, we physicians are baffled: we have no satisfactory medical explanation for why he is still alive.

I have seen other patients go into the operating theater saying that it wasn't going to go well, and though the operation itself was not complicated, it did not go well. I do not know why this happens; no one knows. But over the years, having watched patients get better or get worse, depending on their attitude to what was wrong with them, I have come to believe that there is some mechanism in the brain that has a decisive role in the evolution of certain illnesses.

I suspect that some neurohormonal mechanism must be involved, causing the brain to release greater or smaller amounts of certain hormones according to the person's state of mind, and these hormones modulate the immune system or directly affect other organs, which they reach via the blood.

This is a fascinating field of research, but one in which as yet very little is known for sure. We do not know which illnesses may be influenced by mood, or whether it can prevent or cure them, or if the most it can do is slow their advance, and we do not know how to support and enhance this health-protecting function of the brain. But I believe that some day in the not too distant future we will know the answers.

From Depression to Illness

While we wait for that day to arrive, there are several aspects of the relationship between state of mind and health that we do understand in some detail. More than twenty-five studies of different populations have found that depression increases the risk of premature death. High among the specific diseases to which depressed people are more vulnerable are heart disease and Type 2 diabetes. And it has been found that married people have longer life expectancy than those who live alone, which seems to suggest that the positive emotions of living with a partner have some beneficial effect on health.

Confusion often arises when speaking about depression because the word is used interchangeably to refer to quite different conditions. On the one hand, we often say that someone is depressed when they feel unhappy on account of some negative occurrence such as a family crisis, or losing their job, or the emotional ups and downs that have no obvious cause but almost all of us experience. This type of short-term depression is a natural reaction, and though in extreme cases some form of psychotherapy or drug treatment may be prescribed, it is rarely regarded as an illness.

Then there is another, more persistent, more long-term type of depression, the onset of which sometimes follows a negative personal experience and sometimes seems to be spontaneous, in which there is a malfunction of certain neuron networks in the brain. This is a breakdown in the central computer that plunges the sufferer into an abyss of sadness and pessimism much deeper than transitory depression. And even if you climb out of the abyss, as most of those affected eventually do, it is a condition that, without proper treatment, tends to become chronic.

Though there are significant differences between these two types of depressive disorder, which have to be tackled with different strategies, there are also important points in common. Both are emotional states marked by loss of vitality, dominated by a feeling of having no interest in doing anything. In both there is a tendency to isolate oneself, to shun contact with other people, which tends to have the adverse effect of intensifying the sense of loneliness and sadness. And both have a negative impact on health that goes beyond the psychological distress and affects other organs such as the heart and arteries.

The big question, to which we have only part of the answer, is why depression should have this negative impact. The part of the answer that we know is that negative emotional states lead us to adopt unhealthy behaviors. When you feel depressed, you tend to tell yourself that nothing matters; the despair is so great that you no longer think long term and you stop caring about your health. It is very common, for example, for a depressed person to resort to smoking, drinking, or overeating because these things seem to ease their pain. Depression thus has a negative influence on a number of illnesses in the form of risk factors.

But this does not explain how a patient can survive for more than three years with a cancer that seemed terminal. Nor does it explain why the cardiovascular risk is higher in depressed people even if they do not smoke or drink and are not overweight. So there must be something more, something in a person's state of mind that has a direct influence on health, and that something else is the part of the answer that we do not know. But it is not enough simply to say that depression leads to the disease. To help people, we have to try to understand what happens at the microscopic level, what hormones or other proteins are involved in the cascade of biochemical reactions that lead from depression to disease, which cells these proteins affect, in which organs, whether the immune system is involved or not, whether they produce an inflammatory reaction or not.

If we can understand this whole process in detail, the way we now understand what causes a cancerous cell to multiply uncontrollably, we can develop new therapies to help patients with depression, just as new therapies have been developed in recent years that help cancer patients.

From Happiness to Health

If we know little about the process that leads from depression to disease, we understand even less about how happiness leads to health. When it comes to investigating happiness, one problem is that we have no objective tests with which to diagnose or quantify it, while we do have objective measures for depression. Another problem is that positive states of mind often fluctuate depending on time of day and from one day to the next, whereas depression tends to be more persistent. In addition, since its origins, medicine has been more concerned with investigating diseases in order to cure them than with studying health for the purpose of conserving it, which explains why more effort has been devoted to exploring depression than to understanding happiness.

As a result, we still have no proper scientific studies showing that happiness reduces the risk of any disease. All we have is physicians' day-to-day experience of dealing with patients, which in terms of biomedical research is anecdotal evidence, indicating that happiness and optimism have a positive impact not only on the immediate quality of life but also on long-term health. In my own experience, patients who have a positive attitude are much better at controlling cardiovascular risk factors such as smoking or drinking than those with a negative attitude. They are people who may end up having a heart attack, but because they are optimistic and have confidence in themselves, they do not give up hope, and they do what they have to do to recover.

In other words, a positive state of mind has an indirect influence on health in terms of risk factors, just as depression has an indirect influence on disease. What is less clear, though, is whether there is also a direct influence, by way of hormones, the immune system, or some other biochemical mechanism. A few studies suggest that there is, but they are inconclusive.

For example, a correlation has been established between the positive emotions expressed by a group of nuns in texts they wrote at the age of twenty-two and their subsequent longevity. Another study found a relationship between the degree of satisfaction of members of a large sample of adults in Finland and their survival twenty years later. These are scattered data that suggest a trend but leave us with more questions than answers. Is how happy we are at twenty-two crucial for the rest of our lives, or is the important thing sustaining the state of happiness over several years or decades? What about a person who was unhappy at twenty-two but then sorted out her life, as often happens? And vice versa, what about someone who had been a happy person when he was young but ended up frustrated and bitter, as can also happen? And above all, how much of an impact does happiness have on health? Which hormones, if any, are involved? And which organs are affected?

Laughter, Joy, and Optimism

If we want to get anywhere with our investigation of positive states of mind and understand how they affect health, we must first clarify what we are talking about because, as with depression, the terms we use can be confusing. We all know people who are happy without being cheerful, and others who are cheerful without necessarily being happy. So we will have to analyze separately the effects of joyful gaiety, which is a volatile mood that comes and goes; of happiness, which is more stable and longer lasting, though it may fluctuate according to the time of day and from day to day; of optimism, which is not so much a mood as an attitude; and even of laughter.

My personal impression is that the likely outcome of any thorough research will be to show that long-term well-being and happiness have far more beneficial effects than a relatively short-lived emotion such as joy. And that laughter, which is even more fleeting than joy, probably does not have all the positive effects that have been claimed for it. It has been said that laughter stimulates the cardiovascular system in much the same way as physical activity, that it has a positive impact thanks to the hormones that are released in the brain when we laugh, and there have even been one or two studies in which small groups of volunteers were shown comedy films in order to see whether laughing somehow acts on the endothelium, the inner layer of cells in the arteries.

But the truth is that we do not know what connection laughter has with health, other than that we tend to feel good when we laugh. We simply have no idea what hormonal mechanisms it activates in the brain, or if these have any significant effect on the cardiovascular system.

We know that sick people tend not to laugh very much, but we cannot turn the phrase around and say that a person who laughs a lot will not get sick. I imagine that almost all of us agree that our human ability to laugh is wonderful, one of nature's great blessings. But to go from there to talk about therapeutic properties of laughter is without any scientific basis.

Parrots, Dogs, Cats, and Plants

One piece of advice I give many of my patients who live alone, especially if they feel sad and isolated, is to get themselves a pet. As a rule, I recommend a dog, especially a warmhearted, affectionate breed such as a cocker spaniel, which really shows his feelings and, from what I have seen with my patients, is excellent for lonely people. With a less outgoing, less sociable breed such as the Great Dane or the German shepherd, the patient might not have such a strong sense that their dog is by their side when they feel downhearted.

Keeping a cat can also be very beneficial, but often we tend to form a different kind of bond with a cat than we do with a dog. Cats are more independent, and we are perhaps less likely to feel that we communicate with them. It's not that I don't like cats. On the contrary, we have two cats at home, and one of them is as friendly as a cocker spaniel. But I have found that a dog or a parrot is usually the best pet for a patient who feels alone and downhearted, helping them find more meaning in their life and improving their health.

Often I also recommend a parrot, and though some people are surprised, the overwhelming majority of those who take my advice thank me in due course because parrots fill the house with their chatter and make great company.

It may seem strange for a cardiologist to prescribe a parrot or a spaniel because the way medicine is practiced today, doctors generally confine themselves to prescribing drugs. We physicians increasingly tend to behave like technicians, regarding the patient as an object and treating a heart attack the way an engineer would fix a damaged pump.

But all doctors know deep down that psychological factors have a decisive influence on the origin and evolution of many diseases, and my own experience has shown me that a pet can do more for a patient's health and well-being than any drug. And for those who do not like animals, I recommend plants. This may seem stranger still, but I have seen many patients establish a closer relationship with plants than they would with something inanimate, such as a painting, however beautiful, a TV, a computer, or a car. They water them, clean them, sometimes they talk to them, and the plants grow and change in response to how they are cared for. They are not exactly company, in the way a dog would be, but there is a creative side to caring for plants that many patients find really rewarding.

As for other creative activities such as painting, writing, or playing an instrument, I do not advise against them, but I am not so sure they are of benefit to the patient's health. People who are depressed often feel a need to express their feelings, and there have been many great artists throughout history who have suffered severe depression. But I do not believe that expressing emotions in this way helps a significant percentage of patients to overcome their problems. In any case, it is hard to persuade someone who feels dispirited and has no desire to do anything to summon up the energy and vitality to express themselves creatively.

In fact, a glance at the biographies of depression-prone artists such as Robert Schumann or Tennessee Williams shows that their periods of greatest creativity tend to be times when they were not depressed.

Loneliness and Responsibility

The first thing that getting yourself a dog, a cat, or a parrot does is break the cycle of loneliness, the sense of "no one cares about me, I don't matter to anyone." And of having no one to talk to which is the number one risk factor for alcoholism and causes us to cut ourselves off from others and feel increasingly lonely and negative.

At the same time, and equally important, it puts an end to the feeling of "I don't have anyone to care for" and gives us back a sense of responsibility. People who are depressed very often feel that nothing matters, that it makes no difference whether they take care of themselves or not because when it comes down to it, out there in the world, outside of the shell they have taken refuge in, no one depends on them, so what the hell. But as soon as you have a dog, a cat, or a parrot, there is a living creature that depends on you and that you are responsible for.

This feeling of responsibility is stimulating; it keeps people going and acts as an antidote to depression, helping them stay in control of their lives. From my experience with my own patients, a sense that we are doing something for others, contributing to the community, is vital if we are to feel happy and fulfilled.

People who think only of themselves are extremely vulnerable, and sooner or later they reach a point where they realize that they have done all they can and that there is nothing left for them to do. In part, this explains why the people at the top of the ladder are not, as a group, happier than those of lower social standing.

What Is Success?

Surveys in which people are asked about their material and emotional well-being show no correlation between income and happiness. It is only when people have very little money, not enough to cover basic needs, that poverty emerges as a cause of unhappiness. But above the level of making ends meet, having a newer car, a bigger house, or more expensive shoes does not make us happier. And frequently I find that my working-class patients are happier than the upper-class ones.

It may be worth stopping for a moment to consider whether the scale of values by which social success is measured—the scale of money, power, and fame—corresponds with what we regard as personal success. No doubt some people feel fulfilled by social success. But for others, having time to be with the family on the weekend is more important than having an extra thousand dollars in the bank at the end of the month. So, each of us faces the crucial challenge of defining our own personal scale of values, rather than simply accepting without question the socially "established" scale of values.

I believe that success is about enjoying what you do, knowing you are doing what you ought to, and contributing as much to society as you can: this would be my ideal. It is also about making the most of the good times and not attaching too much importance to the difficult moments because, though the world can sometimes seem like a great big theme park where we can have everything without giving up anything, the fact is that there is no success without some sacrifice, and we all go through tough times and situations that are outside our control.

However, I am not sure that this little emotional survival guide of mine is valid for everyone because we all have our own personal scales of values, and viewpoints, and temperaments.

One thing I am sure of because I see it every day in my office, is that a lot of people have all the social success they want and yet their personal lives are deeply unhappy. And what I always say to them is that social success is irrelevant and that life is short: within a week of your funeral no one will care about who you were, so the best bet is to aim for personal success—to enjoy what you do and help others all you can. And some of them even take my advice.

CHAPTER NINETEEN

At Night

SEX, DRUGS, AND THE HEART

We humans have an amazing knack of worrying about minor threats and paying no attention to the serious ones. Millions of people get anxious about an exotic virus like Ebola, though their risk of being infected is virtually zero, but how many are aware that new antibiotic-resistant strains of *Staphylococcus aureus* cause thousands of deaths in our hospitals each year? There is a public outcry when an outbreak of Legionnaires' disease affects a few dozen people, and certainly the proper measures must be taken to prevent further outbreaks, but hardly anyone seems to care about levels of air pollution that affect thousands.

I come across the same paradox in my office when I see a patient who is concerned about a problem that is objectively minor—though it becomes important from the moment they start worrying about it—and at the same time is paying no attention to problems that are objectively huge.

Misunderstandings About Sex

A typical example of an insignificant problem which causes a disproportionate amount of anxiety is the risk of sexual intercourse resulting in a heart attack. There are plenty of urban myths of people going into cardiac arrest while making love. There are elaborate versions of these stories, embellished with convincing details, in which a man has a stroke in a brothel or in a motel with his lover, and modern versions that wildly inflate the chances of having a heart attack after taking Viagra.

Some elements of these stories are true, but the inference that sexual activity increases the risk of heart attack is false. It is a matter of statistics: there are so many people having sex every minute of every day in every city in the world that it is inevitable that some of them will have a heart attack while making love, just as some will have a heart attack during a business meeting, watching television, or waiting for the bus. But when we look at whether sexual activity has any effect on the risk of heart attack, the influence is negligible.

In other words, the person who has a heart attack while having sex would probably have had it even if they had been sitting on the couch watching TV. And it is as wrong to say that sex increases the risk of heart attack as it is to say that waiting for the bus does. It could be objected that during sexual intercourse, unlike sitting on the couch or waiting at the bus stop, the cardiovascular system is activated in response to the body's need for oxygen and energy and to the partner's demands, all of which means stress for the heart and can have unpredictable results. But this is an exaggeration.

The fact is that many people overestimate the amount of physical activity that sex involves. It has been estimated that, in terms of physical effort, making love is equivalent to climbing two flights of stairs. Just two floors. Which is good news for people who have had a heart attack or have some other heart problem because if they can climb two flights of stairs without getting out of breath or experiencing chest pain, they can resume their sex lives without the slightest fear.

For the same reason—that in most cases it burns off so few calories—it is a mistake to think that sexual activity is as healthy for the heart as real physical exercise. And it has to be admitted that not many couples regularly put in the four sessions a week, of thirty minutes each, that are recommended if physical activity is to produce cardiovascular benefits. There are very good reasons for maintaining an active sex life no matter how old you are: it is gratifying; it is beneficial from an emotional point of view; it is positive for the quality of your relationship with your partner. There are plenty of reasons, all of them very good, but pretending that it counts as physical exercise is not one of them.

Of course, there are couples who put far more energy into their sex life than they would climbing two flights of stairs. But they tend to be couples who both have good cardiovascular health and are perfectly capable of the effort involved in intense physical activity or passionate sexual intercourse. With sex, as with physical exercise, we control our level of activity, and except in special circumstances, such as having had a heart attack in the last four weeks, everyone can do it in a way that they feel is comfortable and safe. So, contrary to popular belief, sexual activity does not have a negative impact on cardiovascular health.

Of far greater concern is the opposite problem, which affects many more people and which gets much less attention: poor cardiovascular health may have very negative effects on sexual activity, especially in men. Atherosclerosis damages the blood vessels which supply the penis and are essential for maintaining an erection, so cholesterol, hypertension, diabetes, and smoking are all front-runners in the impotence stakes. The more cardiovascular risk factors a man has, the greater his chances of ending up with erection problems. And vice versa: the more care he takes over his diet and the more exercise he gets, the lower the risk of impotence in the future.

There has been a good deal of debate about whether the same problem also affects women, and if so, to what extent. Evidently, atherosclerosis also causes deterioration of the arteries that irrigate the genital area in women, especially the clitoris, but it is less clear whether this irrigation is as essential to enjoying sexual activity as it is for men. So, there has been a lot of discussion on this issue, but we do not have sufficient data to assess the scale of the problem, and we have no clear answers. The data we do have suggests that good blood supply to the genital area is also important for women, if they are to enjoy a full sex life, but it is probably less important than it is for men.

Intimate Questions

Even if a person has an exceptionally benign form of atherosclerosis which does not affect the blood supply to the penis or clitoris, many of the drugs we cardiologists prescribe to improve their cardiovascular health—such as beta-blockers, calcium blockers, or statins—can in some cases have side effects that are bad for their sexual health. This is something we physicians must learn to be sensitive to and take the trouble to ask our patients about. For years we tended to neglect the impact of cardiovascular health on a person's sex life, treating it as taboo, and as a result we failed to help many patients in an area of their lives that was very important to them. But now we have begun to talk about the problem more, and we are realizing just how big a problem it is.

Of course, if patients feel unable to tell us, and we feel unable to ask, we are unlikely to find out that a particular drug has affected their sexual capacity and change the treatment, switching to another drug that has no significant side effects. So we doctors have to overcome taboos and learn to ask each patient the relevant questions, respecting their privacy but letting them feel free to discuss whatever it may be that is worrying them.

I recall the case of a fifty-year-old man—an example of a failure of communication between physician and patient. He had suffered a heart attack six weeks before and was eager to move on, eager to resume a normal life, so eager, in fact, that one night he took his partner out to dinner, then took for the first time 100 milligrams of Viagra without having consulted me, and when they got home, they started to make love. Everything was going very well, he said, until it ended suddenly when he passed out.

If he had asked me, or if I had guessed that he would take Viagra so soon after the heart attack, I would not have forbidden it. "Of course you can take Viagra," I would have said. But I would have warned him that as he was already taking several drugs, including some to control hypertension, an excessively large dose of Viagra for the first time could cause a sudden fall in blood pressure, and a lack of blood flow in the coronary arteries and in the brain. Especially when taken just after a big meal, which is what he did because at such times the stomach needs a lot of blood for digestion, and the Viagra will restrict supply to the heart and brain.

So it was okay to take Viagra, but it was not prudent to take it right after a big meal, or to start with 100 milligrams. He ought to have started with 25 milligrams, and if everything went well increase the dose in subsequent times to 50, and then perhaps to 100. And there would have been no problem. The patients who cannot take Viagra are those being treated with nitroglycerin because both drugs dilate the arteries by acting on the nitric oxide and together they can be an explosive cocktail. Nor is it advisable for patients who have low blood pressure and are prone to fainting. But with these two exceptions, any cardiac patient can take Viagra if he does so with proper caution, starting with low doses and with his physician's approval.

Struck Down by Cocaine

The situation with stimulant drugs is the opposite of the situation with sex. Most consumers are unaware that these drugs can damage the heart and have a truly devastating impact (Fig. 1). I have seen patients who have suffered a heart attack at age twenty-five after taking cocaine for the first time. And at thirty. And at thirty-five. I have seen quite a few. And what I have seen is that while it takes cholesterol thirty years of damaging the arteries to bring on a heart attack, cocaine can do it in one night.

Recently in my hospital we analyzed the case of a man of thirty-eight who took alcohol and cocaine one night, came home at dawn, and woke up around noon with a stomach upset. According to his partner, he thought it was gastritis caused by drinking. At two p.m. he was dead. The autopsy a few hours later showed he had had a heart attack. The case strikes me as significant because it makes it clear that, faced with certain symptoms, cocaine users should be aware that they may be suffering a cardiovascular accident.

I do not know how common this problem is. There are no data as to what percentage of occasional cocaine users suffer an immediate cardiovascular accident, or what percentage of habitual users suffer long-term consequences. But I do know that when a person under forty is admitted to the hospital with a heart attack, the chances are that they have taken cocaine. In all likelihood, cocaine, which is a powerful coagulant and also has a tremendous vasoconstrictor effect, has acutely narrowed the arteries and at the same time formed blood clots large enough to block one of the coronary arteries.

Cocaine can also interfere with the electrical system that controls heartbeat and cause sudden death by a rhythm disturbance called ventricular tachycardia. It can cause acute myocarditis, a rare disease in which the heart becomes inflamed and starts beating at top speed.

And it is not only frequent cocaine users who experience these problems. Occasional consumption—in some cases, even taking it just once—can cause devastating damage. But with habitual cocaine abuse the list of possible cardiovascular complications also includes cardiomyopathy, in which the heart muscle deteriorates to the extent that it is unable to pump blood effectively.

We also tend to underestimate the effects of synthetic stimulants such as amphetamines and ecstasy. In the summer of 2005 one of my patients was a twenty-two-year-old who had taken amphetamines for three weeks to help her through her final exams—the academic version of doping—and had ended up with a cardiomyopathy. One of the problems with these drugs is that while not as powerful as cocaine, they tend to constrict the small arteries. Because they are less powerful, it is rare for occasional use to cause a heart attack, though it is not unusual for an overdose of ecstasy to cause anxiety attacks, increased aggressiveness, and even convulsions. But because these drugs have effects similiar to cocaine, repeated consumption, even if only for three weeks, as in the case of the young student, can cause irreversible damage to the heart.

As for the other illegal drugs, there is no evidence that they have a significant effect on cardiovascular health—which does not mean they do not but simply that we do not know if they do or not. When someone smokes marijuana, it is quite possible that the products of the combustion are toxic, not only for the lungs but also for the heart, just as the products of the combustion of tobacco and air pollution are toxic for the heart. And there have indeed been cases of patients who have been habitual marijuana smokers who have developed heart disease. But there is also heart disease among people who have never smoked marijuana, and marijuana smokers who have never developed heart disease, and when we analyze the available data—which is very limited because not much research has been done in this field—it is unclear whether marijuana is a risk factor for heart disease or not.

The Myth of the Full Moon

One thing that is a known factor in the incidence of heart attacks is when they occur. Enough research has been done to give an accurate picture of how heart attacks are distributed according to the time of day, the phase of the moon, and the season of the year, and what it shows is that there are two critical periods in the day when a higher proportion of heart attacks occur. Between six in the morning and midday, the incidence triples, with peak risk in the first hour or two. And between six in the evening and midnight, it almost doubles. By contrast, between midnight and six and between noon and six is when the risk is lowest. That said, even though the risk is statistically lower does not mean we can lower our guard because there are so many heart attacks that they can happen at any time.

No one really knows what causes these changes in incidence during the course of the day. But it is obvious that the human body is adapted to a twenty-four-hour cycle, and that many of the substances that regulate the body's physiology have regular ups and downs throughout the day, such as the melatonin that regulates sleep, the neurotransmitters that regulate hunger, and even the parts of the immune system that regulate fever. So it should come as no surprise that other substances that regulate blood clotting or arterial pressure also go up and down during the day and that this is reflected in an increased risk of heart attack at certain times.

On the other hand, there is no evidence that the level of risk changes significantly with the lunar cycle over the course of the month. The myth that more heart attacks occur at the full moon is just that, a myth, and I do not think it has any more scientific basis than the beliefs of astrology. And it is perfectly logical that the risk should not change throughout the month in the way it changes throughout the day because many of the physiological processes of the human body have a daily cycle, but there is practically no process—with the obvious exception of menstruation—that has a monthly cycle.

As for the annual cycle, there is a relationship with the risk of heart attack: not for any biological reason related to the functioning of the human body but due to cultural causes rooted in the traditions of the particular community. In Christian societies there is an increase in cardiovascular accidents coinciding with Christmas, and in Jewish communities the rise coincides with the end of fasting and the festivities of Rosh Hashanah and Yom Kippur. In my hospital we prepare to receive a greater number of patients when these holidays come around.

Though little real research has been done in this area, I suspect that the increase is due to all the eating and drinking that is done at Christmas, and the consumption of large amounts of very salty foods in the case of the Jewish holidays. Otherwise, there is no significant variation in the risk of heart attack during the year. The risk is pretty much the same come rain or shine, summer heat or winter cold, whether the air pressure is high or low.

Changes in Temperature

For cardiac patients, the problem is not if it is hot or cold, but if the change in temperature is gentle or sudden. I have patients with angina who experience terrible pain when they go from a warm place to a cold place because with the abrupt fall in temperature, their coronary arteries contract and the heart cells are suddenly deprived of oxygen. And I have patients on drugs to control their hypertension who pass out when they go from a cold place to a warm place because the rise in temperature dilates their blood vessels and their blood pressure goes down. So it is generally not a good idea for a cardiac patient to take a sauna. And if you experience chest pain when you come out of the sauna and get under the cold shower, you should see a cardiologist because the pain may be a sign of angina.

Something similar happens with sudden changes in atmospheric pressure, which, incidentally, has nothing to do with blood pressure. Someone with pulmonary hypertension, which affects the blood vessels that carry blood from the heart to the lungs, is very likely to feel bad, with breathlessness or a drowning sensation, if they go up in a chair lift or cable car in the mountains and rise hundreds of feet in a few minutes. People with severe anemia or advanced angina pectoris may also experience discomfort, but this is less common.

The cause, of course, is that the higher the altitude, the lower the atmospheric pressure and the less oxygen there is in the air. In the United States we see the symptoms in people who go to Aspen, Colorado, which is almost 8,000 feet above sea level. And they have also been observed in people who go to Mexico City and develop a pulmonary edema, namely an accumulation of blood in the lungs, at an altitude of over 7,300 feet.

The problem is not high altitude in itself so much as a sudden change in altitude. The same people could visit Aspen or Mexico City without any problem if they traveled up there gradually. With high altitude, just as we said earlier about sex, we can control the level of activity we do and the speed at which we make our ascent, and with the possible exception of those who have breathing difficulties and need to take extra precautions, no one should worry about going to a ski resort or driving over a mountain pass.

CHAPTER TWENTY

Heart Attack

WHEN A CHEST PAIN MEANS YOU SHOULD CALL AN AMBULANCE

No physician I know ever told anyone that went to the emergency room with a suspected heart attack that proved to be a false alarm that they had done the wrong thing. In fact, we find that this is not the case in about 50 percent of the people who come to us thinking they have had a heart attack. And no one should be afraid of looking foolish on account of coming to the emergency room and then finding they have nothing wrong with them. Because the symptoms of a heart attack are not always clear, or particularly painful.

Doctors are well accustomed to seeing patients who think they are dying, and it turns out to be a false alarm; there is nothing ridiculous about it, and we do not find it annoying or feel we are wasting our time making sure that a person is not having a heart attack.

On the contrary, it is a real pleasure to be able to tell someone who comes to you with ambiguous symptoms that they have nothing to worry about and can go home. The person's first reaction is usually to ask: "Are you sure, Doctor?" And when we explain why we are sure, they sometimes apologize for having come. In these cases, I tell them that they have done exactly the right thing because they had symptoms which could have been a heart attack, and other people with similar symptoms have died as a result of not doing what they had the sense to do.

For we physicians, what is really frustrating is not the people who come to the emergency room with what turns out not to be a heart attack but the people who have a heart attack and do not come—and the knowledge that we could have saved 95 percent of the people who die in this way.

This is something that happens every day. I have patients who are Wall Street executives who have called me between two business meetings to tell me they have a pain in their chest. I have been in this situation more than once.

"How long have you had this pain, less than fifteen minutes or more?"

"More than fifteen minutes."

"Does the pain come and go, or is it constant?"

"It's constant."

"When you press your chest, does it hurt more?"

"No."

"Okay, cancel your next meeting, and come over here as fast as possible."

I recall two particular cases where the patient said: "I don't think it's that bad, Doctor, I'll come after the meeting." And it took a great deal of effort to persuade them to come: that what they were describing were the symptoms of a heart attack and their chances of being able to attend meetings in the future were diminishing with every minute that passed, and that if they went ahead with that next meeting, it could well be their last.

Judging from my experience in New York, women tend to be better than men at appreciating the importance of a critical health problem and reacting appropriately to an emergency. I cannot say how true this is of other cultures, but I have often seen men adopt an attitude of denial: they behave as if they were indestructible and refuse to accept that they have a problem even while experiencing the symptoms of a heart attack—like the two executives who were so reluctant to cancel the next meeting.

I simply do not encounter this attitude in women. In fact, I can think of many cases where a woman made her husband go to the emergency room—because he didn't want to come even though he was feeling bad—and her insistence saved his life. On the other hand, I can think of very few cases in which the man persuaded the woman to come to emergency.

Then, once the heart attack has been treated and the patient's life has been saved, it is not uncommon for the man to feel demoralized, disoriented. This is the bewilderment of the person who thought he was invulnerable, who acted the part of a strong, dominant character and now suddenly feels fragile, and no longer knows what his place in the world is. By contrast, women, probably because they acknowledge their vulnerability from the outset, tend to possess more of the emotional strength a person needs if they are going to cope after a heart attack. This is one of the paradoxes one becomes aware of in treating heart patients: the more you accept that you are vulnerable, the less vulnerable you are.

What Is a Heart Attack?

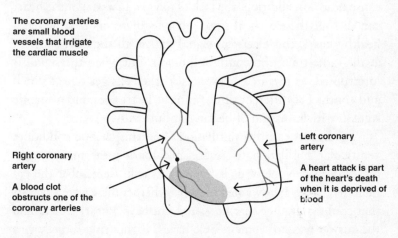

The coronary arteries are small blood vessels that irrigate the cardiac muscle

Right coronary artery

A blood clot obstructs one of the coronary arteries

Left coronary artery

A heart attack is part of the heart's death when it is deprived of blood

Time Is Life

The few minutes after the first symptoms of a heart attack are vital. Of all deaths, 75 percent occur in the first hour from the moment the person realizes that something is wrong. But if they act quickly and get to a hospital, the chance of survival is 95 percent. In other words, out of every 20 patients admitted with a heart attack, 19 are saved. But if we do not act fast, the heart attack runs its course.

The whole drama starts when a blood clot gets stuck in one of the coronary arteries and blocks the flow of blood to part of the heart muscle. When it is starved of blood, and therefore of oxygen, that part of the heart asphyxiates. We physicians call this event tissue necrosis, meaning that the tissue dies. And the heart cells that are destroyed in a heart attack are, in the present state of medical knowledge, irreparable, though current research on stem cells seems to be set to change this in the not too distant future.

This alone, the death of a part of the heart muscle, can be sufficient to put the heart out of action, leaving it unable to pump enough blood to sustain life in the rest of the body and cause death. In addition, the lack of oxygen in a part of the heart can disrupt the electrical signal that regulates its beating. In a healthy heart, this electrical signal makes all the cells contract at the same time, thus pumping blood. But when the signal is interrupted, as it is in a heart attack, the cells get out of synch and contract at different times, and the heart goes into a chaotic state in which, instead of beating, it flutters.

We doctors call this fibrillation. And this chaotic condition, ventricular fibrillation, is responsible for a great many heart-attack deaths. None of us is free of this risk. Remember the patient in chapter 3: he wanted to know whether there were any tests that could guarantee that he would not have a heart attack, and the answer was no. Some people have a higher risk, some have a lower risk, but no one has a zero risk—not even me.

I am a cardiologist, my cholesterol levels and blood pressure are good, I do not smoke, and I get regular exercise, but I could still have a heart attack tomorrow. The statistics show that of every 100 people who suffer a heart attack, about 30 have been previously diagnosed with a heart problem. For the other 70, their first contact with the cardiologist is when they have a heart attack. When we analyze what happened, case by case, we find that about 60 out of those 70 people had known risk factors such as smoking, high cholesterol, or hypertension. But that leaves 10 percent of heart attacks occurring without warning and without the victim having any known risk factor. And then when they ask, "Why me?" we have no answer to give them. We still do not know.

So anyone can be next. And the wisest thing to do, when in doubt, if you are experiencing symptoms that you think may be the onset of a heart attack, is to think the worst and go straight to the emergency room. A heart attack is not the kind of emergency where the person has to wait to be attended to: they get immediate priority. Even if the person is under fifty and has no obvious risk factor, someone with a very low probability of having a heart attack, so much is at stake that the best thing if there is any doubt is to go to the hospital. And we are genuinely delighted if we can say, once we have done all the necessary tests: "False alarm. We are not admitting you. You can go home with an easy mind."

Symptoms to Be Concerned About

But what are the symptoms that should make you suspect you might be having a heart attack? Unfortunately, there is no unequivocal symptom common to everyone who has a heart attack. Some people have one set of symptoms, other people have others, and many of them can be mistaken for symptoms of other problems. The most typical is a pain in the middle of the chest (Fig. 9). This is not just any pain. It is usually crushing: it feels as if someone were sitting on your chest. If it is continuous and lasts for more than fifteen minutes, you should go straight to the emergency room.

And, clearest of all, it is a pain the sufferer will never have experienced before—unless they have had a previous heart attack, in which case they recognize it right away. In some cases, but not in all, the pain may extend to the arms—usually the left—the pit of the stomach, the back, or the jaw. It may not be an unduly intense pain. It used to be thought that the greater the pain, the more acute the lack of oxygen in the heart and the more serious the heart attack. But we now know that this is not the case: a minor heart attack, located in a secondary artery, which affects only a small region of the heart, may be accompanied by tremendous pain, and vice versa; a massive heart attack, with blockage of a main artery and huge destruction of heart tissue, may be accompanied by only mild pain. A heart attack can even be painless.

We estimate that the pain is intense in only about half of all heart attacks. Some 25 percent of people perceive a diffuse pain that they usually do not know what to attribute to. And the remaining 25 percent have no pain. In the absence of pain, there are other symptoms that may also signal the possibility of a heart attack. In the case of the man who had a heart attack after taking cocaine, described in the last chapter, the main symptom was a feeling of indigestion. Other warning signs are nausea, dizziness, or weakness, as well as cold sweats, sometimes accompanied by chest pain and sometimes not: these occur in about half of all heart attacks.

Another symptom, though less frequent, is extreme anxiety and the feeling that one is dying. Or there may be a change in skin color, either pallor or purpleness, especially around the lips. Or a feeling of suffocation because the heart is unable to pump all the blood that reaches it, so that the blood accumulates in the lungs, making it difficult to breathe.

figure 9

PAIN IN AN ANGINA (TRANSITIONAL) AND A HEART ATTACK (LASTING)

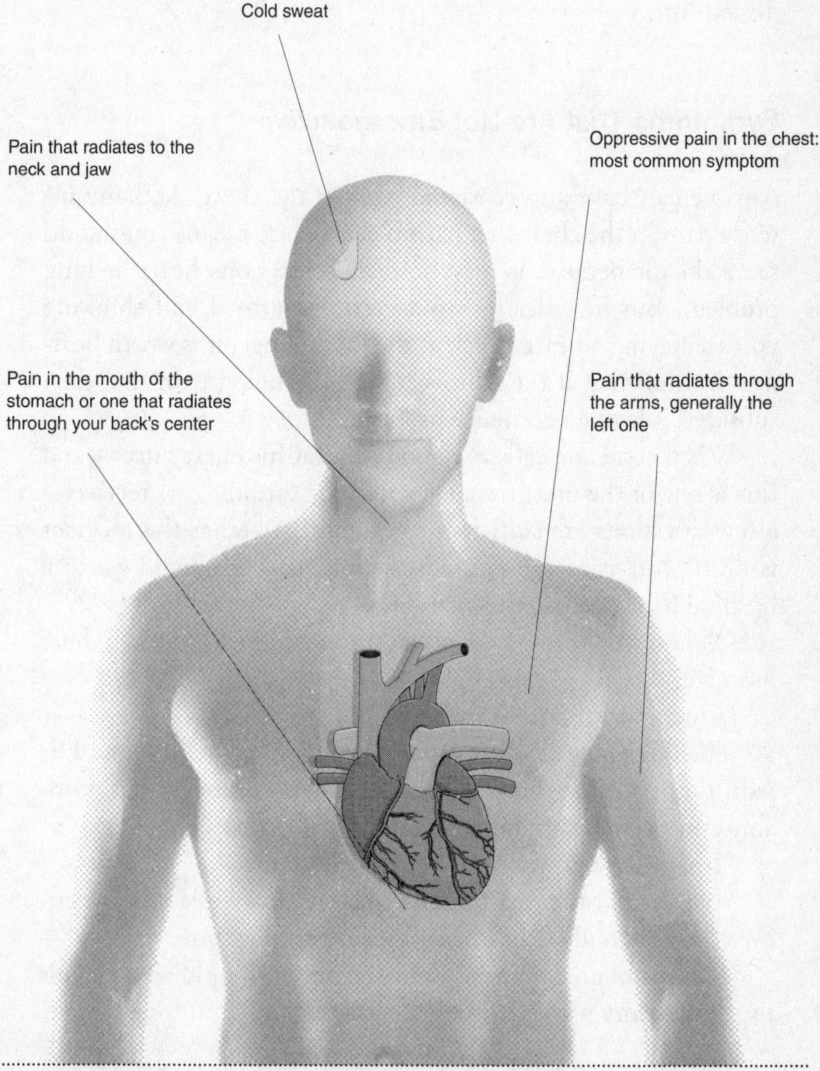

Cold sweat

Pain that radiates to the neck and jaw

Oppressive pain in the chest: most common symptom

Pain in the mouth of the stomach or one that radiates through your back's center

Pain that radiates through the arms, generally the left one

The problem is that all of these symptoms can be due to causes that have nothing to do with the heart. But even if the symptoms are ambiguous, the victim almost always realizes that something out of the ordinary is happening, something they have not experienced before, and given that so much is at stake, it is far better to err on the side of caution and go to the hospital than to ignore the warning signs and dismiss them as temporary discomfort.

Symptoms That Are Not Emergencies

Anyone can have an occasional pain in the chest. And any intense pain in the chest that has no clear cause means you should see a doctor because it may be due to a serious heart or lung problem. But in order to avoid getting alarmed and thinking you are having a heart attack at the first twinge, it is worth bearing in mind that if the pain is sharp, a stabbing pain that then subsides, it is not a coronary problem.

When someone calls me and says that his chest hurts—and this is one of the most frequent calls that cardiologists receive—a few questions are sufficient to establish whether the incident is unimportant or if it could be serious and he should get to a hospital for a proper examination.

"When you press the place where it hurts, does it hurt more?"

"Ouch, yes, it does!"

There is no need for this person to rush to the hospital. His pain is not a heart attack or any other heart problem, but probably comes from the chest muscles.

"Is this the first time you've had this pain?"

"No, it's not the first time. I've had it for a while now, whenever I cough, and lately when I breathe deeply, too."

This is not an emergency, but the person should see a doctor to rule out any possible problem that might affect, for example, the pleura (the membrane that covers the lungs), the pericardium (the membrane covering the heart), or the ribs.

"Is the pain constant or intermittent?"

"It comes and goes. It's a strange pain, as if I was being squeezed. It lasts a minute or two, then goes away, then comes back."

This patient *should* go to the emergency room. Not because they are having a heart attack but because they probably have an unstable angina, which we described before as a pre-heart attack. The pain comes from a partial blockage of the coronary arteries, and 1 in 5 cases will result in total occlusion: in other words, a heart attack in the next five days. When we ask patients who have come to the hospital with a heart attack what they felt in the previous day or two, most say they had an intermittent but generally mild pain in the chest. And many of them had been feeling unwell the day before, or a few hours before, often with nausea or indigestion.

As all of this shows, a heart attack takes place over a number of hours, and the problem is that the most evident symptoms, such as severe pain in the chest or passing out, do not appear until the process is well under way. However, by paying attention to the symptoms that precede the critical phase—the intermittent pain of unstable angina or feeling unwell over several hours, for instance—we can prevent many deaths by intervening before a coronary artery becomes completely occluded.

Lifesaving Defibrillators

When a heart attack has already occurred and the electrical signal that regulates the heartbeats is interrupted, or there is heart stoppage, the best way of saving the maximum number of lives is to have plenty of defibrillators on hand—in shopping malls, sports venues, theaters, stations, airports, even on trains and planes— and train people how to use them. A defibrillator is a device that applies an electrical charge to the heart and restores the signal that causes the cells to contract in synch. In other words, in the event of cardiac arrest, it gets the heart beating again.

For someone who is having a massive heart attack, with blockage of one of the coronary arteries and destruction of a significant amount of heart muscle, there is nothing a defibrillator can do. But for a great many people, surviving a heart attack depends on getting to a defibrillator. Not long ago—this was a textbook case, in which everything went perfectly—a man suddenly collapsed in the stands at a New York Yankees baseball game. He was near the infirmary, and they were able to reanimate his heart with a defibrillator. A few minutes later he was in an ambulance, on his way to the hospital, and they brought him in just thirty minutes after he keeled over in the stands.

We did an electrocardiogram, saw that he was having a heart attack, and injected a thrombolytic drug to liquefy the blood clot. This patient had suffered a heart stoppage so acute that without defibrillation he would probably have died in the stadium. But he was revived so soon, and brought to the hospital so quickly, that when we did another electrocardiogram three days later there was no trace of heart attack. This was remarkable because the characteristic trace left by a heart attack usually shows in electrocardiograms for the rest of a person's life. But in the case of this man, it was as if he had never had a heart attack. His heart was intact. And thanks to the stadium, that there was a defibrillator.

Defibrillators have already saved so many lives that before too long I think it will be the law, or at least common practice, to have them in the places where large numbers of people congregate, such as shopping malls and sports stadiums. They are not difficult to use, but it is essential to have some basic training in order to operate them properly, and I think that in the medium term this training should be given to young people in school, just as they are taught other first-aid and lifesaving techniques.

In the United States, people with a major risk of heart

attack—people who have already had one and whose cholesterol or blood pressure is still too high—often now have their own defibrillator at home and teach their family how to use it. I have patients who are alive today thanks to a home defibrillator, and I feel sure that in the not too distant future insurance companies will pay for them. They are still expensive—the price of a unit starts at about $1,500 and goes up to over $5,000, and some of those bought are never used—but they are cheap compared to the value of a person's life.

Upon Arriving at Emergency

The first thing we do when someone is brought into the emergency room with a suspected heart attack is to run an electrocardiogram and give them a dose of sublingual nitroglycerin, a tablet placed under the tongue where it dissolves and passes into the bloodstream. The electrocardiogram shows if there is a blood-flow problem anywhere in the heart. The nitroglycerin, which instantly dilates the arteries, tells us if the problem is an unstable angina or a heart attack. With an unstable angina, the pain disappears in a minute or so because the coronary arteries dilate and normal blood flow is restored. With a heart attack, the pain does not go away because nitroglycerin cannot dissolve the clot and blood flow remains blocked (Fig. 9).

We next give the patient a dose of aspirin, which helps prevent further clots from forming, and if the diagnosis of heart attack is confirmed, we come to the critical moment when we have to decide how to restore circulation in the blocked coronary artery. We have three options: angioplasty with stenting, drugs, or bypass. And hardly any time to think.

The first option is angioplasty or a stent (Fig. 10). With no need for anesthesia, a catheter is inserted in the thigh and fed through the arteries to the heart. When it reaches the point where the heart attack has occurred, a small balloon is inflated to open up the occluded artery by pressure from inside—this is what we call angioplasty—and a small mesh tube, what we call a stent, is implanted to stop the artery closing again. Within fifteen minutes or so, blood flow is restored.

Of the various options available to us at present, this is the best: no other is faster or more effective or safer. The problem is that not every health center has a catheterization unit with staff trained to unblock a coronary artery. If the patient was more than two hours from a hospital with a catheterization unit when the heart attack occurred, and is admitted to a small county hospital shortly after the onset of symptoms, then the best option is to start removing the clot with drugs (thrombolytic therapy, Fig. 10). In these first two hours, drugs are about as effective as angioplasty. They can cause hemorrhaging, however, though we now have that risk fairly well under control, and it may still prove necessary to implant a stent a few hours or a few days later.

As for coronary artery bypass, these days this technique is used less than it was a few years ago because it is more aggressive, but not more effective, than a stent. This is a surgical procedure in which a non-vital piece of vein or artery is taken from another part of the patient's body and grafted into the heart (Fig 10). The graft, just a few centimeters long, connects the aorta and the coronary artery, forming a bridge across the section of blood vessel that has been occluded, thus restoring circulation. This is a very effective technique in chronic heart patients, but in acute cases it is now usually confined to the minority of patients that cannot have a stent or have had an implant that has failed.

Once the critical stage is past, and the coronary artery is functioning again, the patient will probably be kept in the hospital for about three days—between two and five days, as a rule. Before he or she is discharged, we have a very important meeting where we talk about their lifestyle, their risk factors, and how they can prevent another heart attack. We generally prescribe four drugs: aspirin (because it is anti-inflammatory and anti-coagulant), a statin (for its anti-inflammatory and cholesterol-

figure 10

CORONARY INTERVENTIONS

Catheter   Inflated balloon   Obstructed artery

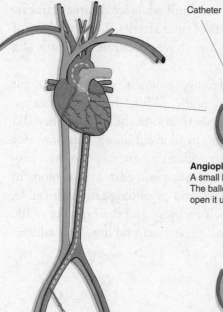

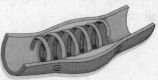

Angioplasty
A small balloon-tipped catheter reaches the heart. The balloon inflates within the coronary artery to open it up by adding pressure.

Stent
A metal or plastic mesh tube (stent) can be implanted within the artery to avoid future blockage.

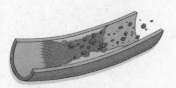

Thrombolytic Therapy
If no more than two hours have passed since the initial heart attack symptoms, thrombolytic medicine could help break up the clot and reestablish circulation within the obstructed artery.

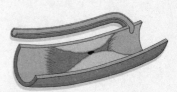

Bypass
A fragment of another one of the patient's vein is joined together and bridged over the obstructed area of the coronary artery so that the blood can go around the obstruction and keep circulating regularly. The bypass connects the aorta with the obstructed artery.

reducing effects), a beta blocker (which helps the heart consume oxygen more efficiently and reduces the risk of another heart attack), and what we call an ACE inhibitor (which keeps the heart from deteriorating further in the days after the heart attack).

We also ask some people to do a low-intensity stress test, in which they run slowly on a treadmill while we do an electrocardiogram and analyze the state of their arteries. The sensitivity of the test may be increased by the above procedure by means of a special imaging technique.

And then comes the decisive moment, when the patient leaves the hospital and goes home. While they were with us, we treated them to the very best of our ability, and they did not have to decide what to do or to avoid doing. But now, day 3 after the heart attack, they suddenly have to adapt to a new situation, a situation they had not planned for, at a moment when they are physically weak and psychologically vulnerable. It is day 3 of a new life. Their recovery and their quality of life in the future will depend to a great extent on how they address this critical time.

CHAPTER TWENTY-ONE

After a Heart Attack

MAKING A NEW START

Sometimes I wonder how I would react if I had a heart attack. I do not mean how I would react in the first few minutes, crippled with chest pains and a debilitating feeling of sickness. If the symptoms are clear, I think I would know how to spot them and unless I died on the spot, I think I would get to the hospital on time. I mean how I would react later, after getting out of the hospital, from day 3 of my new life. And the truth is I'm not sure.

A part of me says I would handle it well—that I would know how to move on without blaming myself for whatever wrong I might have done to my health, or sinking into depression, or living in the grip of fear of suffering another heart attack. I think I would know how to go back to leading a normal life. And if the heart attack were bad enough to damage my heart to the extent that I could no longer cycle over mountains in the Pyrenees and the Alps as I like to do, I think I would be capable of finding other activities to fulfill myself. Because, in the end, that is what responding well to a heart attack means: being able to move on, regardless of how debilitated you might be.

But I have seen so many cases of people who seemed so strong-willed—high-ranking politicians or corporate executives who make 100-million-dollar decisions—but then crumbled after a heart attack, and I have seen so many cases of people that seemed weak-willed but then showed remarkable fortitude that I have come to the conclusion that it is impossible to predict how anyone will react. My personal impression is that the people who deal with it best are the ones who take a more realistic view of life and their place in the world, who do not overestimate their own strength and accept a heart attack as one of the risks they run.

But a heart attack triggers such deep-rooted emotional reactions, reactions that are tough to handle in a rational manner, such as fear of dying or the feeling that youth has abruptly ended, that there is really no way to know how someone will react until they actually have a heart attack.

Three Ways to React

In the three days a heart attack victim normally spends in the hospital, his entire world changes. When he comes into the emergency room on Monday, we have a heart attack to deal with and we give the same fast and direct treatment we give in any similar case. But on Thursday, when we discharge him, we are no longer dealing with an illness but with a person filled with doubts, fears, and physical weakness: a person for whom life just took an unexpected turn. Now we have no quick, direct fixes: we must employ far more subtle means. The same treatment, the same counseling, does not work for everyone. Nonetheless, although every person reacts differently, after dealing with patients for more than thirty years, I believe post-heart attack attitudes can be divided into three main groups.

About a third of patients take a positive attitude, seeing their heart attack as a sign that something was wrong in their lives and making the decision to fix it. I have even had a few patients whose families or friends ended up saying: "You're so lucky you had a heart attack!" Because later on, when they begin to take care of themselves, they feel much better and get more out of life.

Another third take the opposite turn, down Pessimism Street, and fall prey to depression. They feel defeated, emotionally devastated, sometimes without a clear idea of what life holds for them now. And the big challenge we have as doctors in these cases is to steer them off a path that inevitably leads them down a dead-end street.

Finally, what marks the other third is fear. They are so afraid of having another heart attack that they do not dare to lead a normal life. They could drive but prefer not to. They could have sex but refrain. They could go on a vacation overseas—but what if their heart gives out on them so far from home? They are so cautious that they end up leading a limited life of petty restrictions they impose upon themselves. In such cases, what we have to do is to restore their confidence so that they dare to venture out and face the real world again.

What you almost never see is a "so-what?" attitude. For anyone that has one, a heart attack means a change of plans, in many cases even a complete change in lifestyle, and it obliges you to adapt to a new situation you never anticipated. And everyone, from the optimist to the pessimist and the frightened, faces the same two problems.

On the one hand, you face the physical problems of having atherosclerosis that will require treatment and living with a weakened heart that might never regain the strength to pump blood as effectively as before. And then there are the psychological problems associated with heart attack: feelings of guilt, of being dependent on others, and, often for the first time in life, of being vulnerable and mortal.

How to Help Someone Who Has Had a Heart Attack

The doctor is in the best position to help a heart-attack victim deal with their physical problems. After discharge, before our first monthly appointment, I usually phone my patients. I do this because it is a key moment in their recovery, a moment on which their future depends, and it is positive for them to know that their physician has not forgotten about them. They need to know that their doctor cares whether they are taking their medication and following recommendations. They need to know their doctor is willing to answer any questions they have and that they can call whenever they like, and that their doctor will help them to recover as best he or she can.

But the doctor's support must not be paternalistic because if they treat the patient like a child or a dependent, the patient is likely to end up developing a dependence, sometimes even to the point of hypochondria. Dependent patients ask countless questions about minor issues and see their doctor as a source of security, as a father-like figure rather than as a physician, a situation that impedes them from regaining their autonomy.

The same goes for the family, who can be a great help in overcoming the psychological scars of a heart attack. But what family should never do is to make the common mistake of treating the patient as if they had ceased to be an independent person. The "I'll watch your diet for you" attitude, which is a very common reaction, often leads to food obsessions and feelings of guilt or blame regarding minor issues such as one day having a steak rather than grilled sole.

Another common error, also counterproductive, is the "I told you so" attitude. After a heart attack people usually suffer enough guilt feelings about everything they did wrong with their health, and the last thing they need from a spouse or child is a scolding—what they do need from them is support. Nor should family, worried about the risk of another heart attack, transmit their anxiety or fuss about whether the patient is taking care of himself, eating right or taking his meds because this will not help him overcome his own anxiety.

So what can the family do to help? Above all, support the patient to resume a normal life, if possible life as it was before the heart attack, free from pressures, respecting their doubts and fears. Suggest getting out of the house, going to the movies, exercising together outdoors, going away for the weekend: in short, the "why don't we take that trip to Paris" attitude. And—one of the things I say always to my patients—move on!

"I'm Going to Live Right from Now On"

After a heart attack, the people who find it easiest to cope are those who take a positive attitude: they realize that the life they were leading was unsustainable and are willing to change. This attitude does not depend on the size of their heart attack. There are people who suffer a massive heart attack with major damage to their heart but nevertheless adopt a positive attitude, and there are people who suffer a relatively minor heart attack with barely any permanent damage but then sink into despair.

A positive attitude need not be immediate. I recall a recent case (very typical, by the way) of a man—fifty-eight years old, smoker, obese, hypertension, a completely disorganized life—who suffered a heart attack. The tests we did before discharging him showed he had had a medium-sized attack and that there was not too much damage to his heart. He went home with our prescriptions and advice, convalesced for a few days (reflecting on his life, I imagine), and then returned to his management position in a communications company. When I saw him again a month later, I could see he was very worried. He felt unable to keep up with the pace of his job and felt that the world around him was falling apart.

Then I suggested that this might be a great opportunity to change his life, which until then had been erratic, and to start to take care of himself and discover new pleasures. And his reaction could not have been more positive. He said: "Doctor, the time I have left to live, and I don't know if it will be long or short, I assure you will be good; my life is going to be better from now on." So a month after his heart attack, he changed his attitude and started to take care of himself. But what happened then with this patient is a pattern I have seen in others and illustrates the major pitfall of such a positive attitude.

As usual, we had our next appointment scheduled for six months after the heart attack. But he called a few days earlier to say he could not make it because he had a meeting too important to miss. We rescheduled him for another day, and a few days before that appointment, he called again. This time he had a business trip he could not cancel. We scheduled a third appointment, which he postponed due to some family problem. In the end, I did not see him again until over a year after the heart attack.

He had started smoking again; he had stopped exercising, gained weight, and gone back to his poor eating habits. He had felt so good after starting to take care of himself that he thought he had beaten his health problems and as a result resumed all the bad habits that had led to his heart attack in the first place.

This is the great paradox of such patients: if they believe they have beaten it, they are bound to lose; if they are aware they can lose, then they are bound to win. And what we doctors must do in these cases is encourage them to continue to take care of their health and to temper their enthusiasm, while reminding them that although they might feel better than ever, they still rank high in risk of another heart attack.

Patients Who Become Depressed

With patients who sink into a cycle of depression, we have to take the very opposite tack: instead of stressing the risk of another heart attack, doctors must play it down. This is not meant to mislead the patient, denying that he had a heart attack or that he may have another. But if you feel psychologically devastated after having a minor heart attack, you need to know that it was small and that your chances of recovery are excellent if you follow our advice.

If the heart attack was major, you need to know that you will feel much better if you watch your diet, exercise, and quit smoking—and that by doing so you can avoid another heart attack. And for the person who led a healthy life before having a heart attack but has a genetic predisposition to atherosclerosis—a difficult case because they feel they have done everything possible, all for nothing—it is worth recalling that today we have new drugs and know a lot more about how to treat heart attack victims, and that their life expectancy can be as long as other people's.

It is not unusual for a depressed patient to break down and cry in the doctor's office. And from my experience, the best thing you can do to help them to cope is to make them see the positive side of their recovery. Nor is it uncommon for a patient, after seeing the cardiologist for his heart, to see a psychiatrist for his depression, and for the psychiatrist to prescribe an antidepressant. And while there are situations where antidepressants can be helpful, I believe they are a minority. Personally, in these cases I have much more faith in the doctor-patient relationship than I do in drugs because we are not dealing with depression caused by a malfunctioning of the brain—in which case drugs may well help—but with a mental type of depression spurred by the patient's thoughts as a result of a heart attack. Even if you give him antidepressants, he will still know he had a heart attack.

So the best way to get to the root of the problem is to talk to the patient and make him see that he has only a partial view of what is happening: that it is true that his heart has been damaged and, yes, that is bad, but that there is a lot of life after a heart attack and that he has the chance to enjoy it just as much as anyone else.

Fear of Another Heart Attack

As for the fearful type of patient, who is likely to have a hard time getting his life back on track, we must ask ourselves how we can help him to restore his courage. Such patients impose a lot of restraints on their lives, avoiding activities they could do but do not feel capable of.

A strategy I find often works with these people is simply to tell them to walk a mile a day. When they realize they can do that, they regain confidence in their physical capacities and are soon walking longer and longer distances, until one day they try running. Moreover, if the heart attack was minor, light exercise like walking has the advantage of requiring no medical supervision, which helps them feel independent again.

On the other hand, in the case of a major heart attack, the patient should begin exercising under a supervised rehabilitation program, where it is harder to restore a sense of independence and self-confidence. When someone loses a third of their viable heart muscle and slips into a cycle of fear, they may even become afraid to walk because it makes their heart beat faster, and it is not enough to stress the positive side of recovery as with depressed patients. From my experience the best approach for someone in this situation is to explain from the outset that their lives will never be like before, that their heart has lost part of its ability to pump blood, but from now on we are going to work together to improve their quality of life.

And what I've learned in dealing with such difficult cases is that people have a tremendous capacity for overcoming their problems, and even when a problem is so daunting that coping seems impossible, we can tackle it by dividing it into smaller problems and addressing them one by one: walk 100 meters today, 110 tomorrow, and in the end a person can again lead a relatively normal life in spite of having suffered a massive heart attack.

Mission: Return to Normal Life

A heart attack is not necessarily a sentence to early death. Statistics show that 5 percent to 6 percent of heart attack victims have another heart attack within three months, with maximum risk in the first six weeks, after being discharged from the hospital. Following these critical three months, the risk goes down to 2 percent to 3 percent a year—that is, for every 100 people that have already had a heart attack, each year two or three will have another, and in ten years more than twenty will. Which also means that over those same ten years nearly 80 percent will remain heart attack free, and there are people who tackle their health problems, control their cholesterol and blood pressure, and live to see their ninetieth birthday and beyond, way over the average life expectancy. That's why it's so important for everyone to follow their doctor's advice and take their medication: it's your ticket to a long, fulfilling life.

But physicians must recognize that too often we are unable to convince our patients to do as we tell them: just one year after a heart attack, nearly 50 percent of victims already relax and no longer follow all of their physician's advice, which is an extremely high rate of failure. Where we fail most is with medication: many people simply find it hard to follow a regimen that normally includes no fewer than four different drugs, and sooner or later they begin to grow lax. Sometimes they feel so well they act as if they had never had a heart attack and stop taking their drugs altogether. Or they feel so depressed they do not care. Or they simply forget to take them. In the end, for one reason or another, most patients fail to follow their treatment.

By following the doctor's advice and keeping up with medication, there is no reason why the life of a heart-attack survivor should be much different from that of any healthy person, especially if the heart attack was minor. Patients often ask me: "Doctor, can I still work like I did before?" Of course you can: a heart attack does not mean you have to give up your job. I have patients who are judges, and even working under all that pressure, they have gone back to work without a hitch. "Will I be able to ski again?" Yes, you can: you can ski or do any other aerobic exercise such as swimming, tennis, or cycling; only when a stress that the heart suffers with such activities—less than of all cases—do we recommend that the patient wear er and not exceed a certain pulse rate. And then there question that most concerns patients, the subject they are most afraid to broach, so if they do not ask, I do: "Can I have an active sex life like before?" And the answer is yes, you can.

So, given some patients' tendency to look back, to feel psychologically chained to a heart attack that happened some time ago, I often remind them that each life is a project permanently under construction. The idea that for each person there is only one possible path, and that if we get hit by a heart attack or some other accident along the way, we derail and can no longer arrive at our destination, strikes me as being utterly mistaken.

In reality, each life is the sum of manifold variables and circumstances, and a heart attack can be one of those variables but is not necessarily the most important one. And even if a heart attack damages your heart so badly you will not be able to do certain activities, surely you can find other equally rewarding activities. You live your life as you decide to live it, I remind patients. And the best advice I can give is: *move on*.

CHAPTER TWENTY-TWO

Stroke

AN EMERGENCY MORE URGENT THAN A HEART ATTACK

Despite heart attack's bad reputation, with all its seriousness, there is another type of atherosclerosis-related emergency that is even worse: stroke, or cerebrovascular accident, in which a brain artery becomes blocked or bursts and millions of neurons are destroyed. It's worse for doctors because diagnosing the problem in order to determine the correct treatment is more complicated than with a heart attack, while the time window to act is narrower. And above all, it is worse for the patient because stroke often results in some sort of permanent disability. That is why so many patients and colleagues in the medical profession have told me that the last thing they want to have is a stroke. They can handle a heart attack because it leaves the brain intact and you can get over it. But a stroke they dread because they fear being incapacitated and do not want their families to be forced to care for them.

Different Kinds of Stroke

The first problem we face when someone comes into the emergency room with symptoms of a stroke is that there is no way to tell at first glance exactly what has happened, and the most effective treatment in some cases is harmful in others. If someone comes in with a myocardial infarction, there is no doubt what has happened And it's easy to decide what to do, but a stroke can be one of three different things.

First, it could be an embolism: an occlusion of the arteries that supply blood to the brain caused by a clot that originated elsewhere in the body and "rafted" through the bloodstream to the brain. These clots that travel through the blood, and that often come from the cavities of the heart, the carotid arteries in the neck, or the aorta, we call emboli (singular: embolus), hence the name embolism.

A stroke may also be what we call an in situ thrombus: the blockage of an artery in the brain caused by a clot formed in the same artery. Clots that form inside blood vessels are called thrombi, and they can either break loose or remain embedded where they form—unlike clots that form to repair the walls of veins and arteries after an injury, or those that form on skin cuts. Hence the name thrombosis, which is the abnormal formation of clots inside blood vessels, or in this case, in situ thrombus, meaning that the clot forms at the same point where it causes damage.

Finally, a stroke can mean a brain hemorrhage, in which a brain artery ruptures and blood that spurts out under pressure floods a part of the brain. Anyone that has had a broken pipe at home can get an idea of how far and fast fluid—blood in the case of a brain hemorrhage—can spread when under high pressure. And anyone who has ever had a good bruise has an idea of the damage a discharge of blood can cause to neighboring tissues.

In the first two types of stroke—embolism and in situ thrombus—an artery is occluded, cutting off the blood supply to part of the brain. Both are what we call a cerebral infarction because the infarction occurs due to the occlusion of an artery, as in a myocardial infarction, or heart attack.

In a cerebral hemorrhage the opposite happens: instead of drought, we have a flood. Paradoxically some brain hemorrhages are due to the occlusion of an artery, which bursts after being blocked by a thrombus. This latter case is known as a hemorrhagic infarction.

Opposite problems call for opposite solutions. In occlusive strokes the idea is to get the blood flowing again. With a hemorrhage, ideally, in the spot where the injury has occurred, you have to stop the flow.

The Three Big Types of Ictus
In an ictus, or stroke, a massive destruction of neurons is produced because of the obstruction or bursting of a blood vessel in the brain.

1 Embolism
A blood clot coming from another organ, transported by the blood, arrives and obstructs a brain artery.

2 Thrombus
A blood clot forms within a blood vessel in the brain and obstructs it.

3 Brain Hemorrhage
A blood vessel bursts in the brain and floods the neighboring tissue with blood.

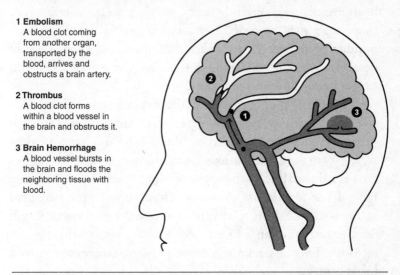

But although the problems are different, the damage is the same. In all types of stroke there is a decimation of neurons, neurons that are lost forever because brain cells, unlike those of other organs, rarely regenerate; however, if they do regenerate, then they do so poorly and the victim is no longer able to do the things the dead neurons once controlled: things as basic as speaking or walking, or using your right hand, suddenly become impossible.

The specific damages suffered by an individual stroke victim depend on the part of the brain that has been destroyed: it can affect sight if the vascular accident occurs at the rear of the brain, where the neurons that control vision are located; it can cause paralysis in half the body if it occurs in the front of the brain; it may affect balance if it happens near the ear. The sort of damage varies widely, but if the stroke is big enough, it is almost always serious, and the odds of full recovery are virtually nil.

Tomorrow Is Too Late

Although they have traditionally received less attention than heart attacks, and certainly many people have less awareness of them than they have of heart attacks, strokes cause a similar number of deaths. Heart attack remains the leading cause of death in Western countries. But strokes come a close second, cancer being almost as prevalent.

The main problem is that the brain is a terribly sensitive organ, whose neurons deteriorate faster than the cells of the heart when deprived of blood, and the time window we have to save the patient from the moment a stroke occurs is minimal. If in the event of a heart attack we generally have up to four hours to restore circulation to the occluded artery—although in relatively rare cases, a heart attack will require faster action—in a stroke we have two to three hours at most. Thus a stroke is a more pressing emergency than a heart attack.

An added problem is that when a stroke victim gets to the hospital, before deciding what action to take, doctors must first clarify whether they are dealing with an occlusion or a hemorrhage. In a heart attack, as soon as the victim arrives, all efforts are directed at removing the clot blocking the coronary artery. But in a stroke you cannot immediately administer a thrombolytic drug to dissolve a potential clot because if it is a hemorrhage—and there is a 15 percent chance of it being so—the drug would only aggravate the situation.

So the first thing to do is to examine the patient with a computed tomography, an imaging technique with which you can see the status of the arteries, and in most cases you have the results in twenty minutes. If computed tomography is not available and the patient is examined with an MRI, the result may be delayed for all of forty-five minutes. If, in addition, the hospital is not equipped to deal with such emergencies, as still happens in some hospitals where there are no neurologists permanently assigned to the emergency room, or where there are computed tomography machines but they are in another department, even more time is lost. And for every minute that goes by, the less chance there is of saving the patient from suffering major disabilities for life.

When you finally get a diagnosis, it's time to act. If imaging techniques reveal an embolism or an in situ thrombus, a thrombolytic drug called tPA is administered, which usually restores circulation to the occluded artery but can cause brain hemorrhages and should be administered only within the first three hours after the onset of symptoms. Beyond three hours, the risks of the drug outweigh the benefits.

In cases where the diagnosis is a hemorrhage, we have no drug that can save the patient, although in some cases we have the option of transferring them to the operating theater and draining the stagnant blood off the brain.

All in all, once everything possible has been done, approximately three out of four stroke survivors are left some sort of permanent damage that can range from minor to devastating.

Three out of four is a poor record and shows that we are treating too many patients too late. And when one wonders why the result is so poor, part of the answer is that a stroke wreaks havoc almost immediately, and no matter how fast you act, it will always be difficult to arrive on time. Another part of the answer is logistics: the health system is not equipped to meet such emergencies as quickly as required, although progress is being made to address this problem. Another part is technical: we have fewer drugs to deal with a stroke than we have to treat a heart attack, for example.

But there is still another aspect of the problem in which what doctors do and the means available to them have no direct bearing: rather the problem lies with stroke victims themselves and their families. Too many people do not know how to recognize the early symptoms of a stroke and they react late.

In the United States most patients take more than twelve hours to go to the ER from the moment they begin to notice that something is wrong with them. A common mistake occurs when an elderly member of the family suffers some symptom of a stroke, such as a slight speech impediment or partial paralysis of a limb, which is not always accompanied by a feeling of being ill. "Let's wait and see how he is tomorrow. If he's not any better then, we'll take him to the hospital," the family may say. And when they get him to the hospital the next day, it's too late.

How to Recognize a Stroke

So what are the signs that someone may be having a stroke? In some cases, especially with an embolism or hemorrhaging, they are very evident. The person tries to speak but cannot make themselves understood or cannot understand what others say; or half the face twists; or part of the body is paralyzed; or it might be that they cannot pick up a pencil or a glass because they lack the strength in one hand; or they cannot see out of one or both eyes; or they may even fall to the floor because they do not have the strength to stand. Any of these signs is possible, although not all at once because it depends on the area of the brain that has been damaged, and any one of them is cause for an immediate visit to the emergency room, even if the person says they feel okay and does not want to go.

One obstacle to early diagnosis is precisely that a stroke does not typically cause pain or discomfort, although in a minority of cases the first symptom is a bad headache, and people are liable to think nothing is wrong with them when in fact their life is hanging by a thread.

In other cases, the signs are less obvious, although the vascular accident may be just as serious. In an in situ thrombus, for example, the symptoms tend to appear more gradually than in an embolism or hemorrhage. A few hours, or even a few days before the actual stroke, one may begin to notice a loss of motor control in one hand or that the tongue cannot pronounce certain letters, or a feeling of unsteadiness when walking. This usually happens because the thrombus is still forming and gradually cuts off the blood flow before a total occlusion occurs. In an embolism, however, the flow is blocked abruptly at the moment when the embolus is lodged in the artery, so the signs likewise appear suddenly.

On the other hand, if instead of affecting the areas of the brain that control body movement or speech, the stroke affects areas involved in memory or reasoning, it is likely that the early warning signs will go unnoticed. You may sense that something is not right but you cannot quite figure out what it is; or you might realize what it is but keep quiet about it, while the people around you do not notice anything wrong with you.

And the people around you often play a decisive role in identifying the early symptoms of a stroke and in convincing you to go to the hospital. It is not uncommon for people to be completely unaware of what is happening to them: they keep trying to talk without realizing that no one can understand them, or they keep trying to walk without realizing that part of their body is failing to respond to their brain signals.

And in such cases it is the people around the stroke victim who must seize the initiative and say: "We're taking you to the hospital." And if the victim replies, "The hospital, what for?" as sometimes happens, they must insist until they convince him.

What to Do If the Signs Let Up

It may be that the symptoms of a stroke disappear after a few minutes or a few hours: when grandfather went to bed he could not move his leg, but the next morning it was moving again. So the family thinks: "We were right to wait and see what a bit of sleep would do; there's no need to take him to the hospital after all." And they are making a big mistake.

What actually happened to this man was not some insignificant ailment that goes with old age, as the family thinks, but what we call a transient ischemic attack. We call it ischemic—a brief explanation for those readers who are beginning to acquire a taste for medical jargon—because it is caused by a cerebral artery stroke and it produces an ischemia, in other words a local deficiency of blood supply. And we call it transitory because it resolves itself spontaneously when the thrombus that occluded an artery disintegrates and the flow of blood is restored.

Once the blood is flowing again, significant repercussions are rare and the most common reaction is to believe that it was nothing, a minor incident without consequences. But such a reaction is wrong: like a small earthquake that causes no damage, a transient ischemic attack may be the prelude to a catastrophic event. To put it in numbers, 5 percent—1 in 20—of those affected by a transitional attack suffer a major stroke within three months. After one year, the percentage rises to 14 percent—1 in 7. And after ten years the rate is almost 50 percent, or 1 in 2.

So, in the event of any transient ischemic attack, no matter how brief, no matter how minor the signs, you should see a neurologist within the next few days to avoid having a major incident. Even more frequent than transient ischemic attacks are what we call microembolisms, the occlusion of small blood vessels in the brain, which causes a small but significant loss of mental faculties and physical abilities. Microembolisms are a common problem in older people and are usually diagnosed by doing an MRI scan of the brain. They require medical treatment, not so much to repair any damage, which may be irreversible, as to prevent further microembolisms or a major stroke.

A Disaster That Can Be Prevented

For years we accepted strokes as inevitable,, an unfortunate occurrence that struck without warning, and against which there was little doctors could do. But medical science has advanced far enough—the development of magnetic resonance or tPA, for instance—that today we can not only treat but prevent many strokes.

The most important preventive measure is to control blood pressure, hypertension being the number one risk factor in stroke and even more of a threat to the brain than to the heart. Blood coagulability should also be monitored—if your blood clots too easily there is a propensity for thrombi to occur, while low coagulability can lead to hemorrhage. It is also important, of course, to watch your cholesterol, which lies at the root of a high percentage of vascular accidents, both in the brain and in other organs.

A large part of stroke prevention is in the patient's hands: you can lower your odds of having a stroke by much the same means as you can lower your odds of a heart attack: watch your diet, exercise, don't smoke, and keep an eye on your blood pressure.

But here, prevention depends to a greater extent, far greater than with heart attacks, on doctors and on the health care system. Only doctors can determine the best treatment in cases of hypertension. And only we can prescribe the right anticoagulants to lessen the risk of embolism or in situ thrombus without increasing the risk of hemorrhage.

Doctors can identify the origin of the clots that cause transient ischemic attacks. If the clot comes from, for example, one of the carotid arteries—which run up either side of the neck to the brain—we can determine whether the artery is severely narrowed and whether an angioplasty to dilate it and restore blood flow is in order.

In theory, all of this is within our realm of possibilities, and prevention has improved in recent years, thanks mainly to advances in the treatment of hypertension. But still the reality is that too many people have strokes that could be prevented with what we know today.

Life After a Stroke

When prevention fails, the probability of surviving a stroke stands at 85 percent, better odds than with a heart attack, where the survival rate is around 70 percent. But only a minority of the people who survive a stroke suffer only minor or no permanent damage, whereas the vast majority of heart attack survivors can go back to leading a perfectly normal life.

Among stroke victims, the "move on" attitude we spoke about in regard to a heart attack, the "I'm-going-to-start-taking-care-of-myself" attitude, is unusual. Even for the most optimistic person, the emotional blow from having a part of your body paralyzed, or wanting to speak and not being able to, can be overwhelming. And the fear of another vascular accident, which is a common reaction after a heart attack, is seen in few patients.

For the family, too, who suddenly have to reorganize their lives to care for a person who can no longer fend for themselves, the impact of a stroke is enormous.

Patients usually experience a noticeable improvement in the first few days as the body eliminates the fluid that accumulated in the brain during the vascular accident. But six months later, according to a study done in the United States, 50 percent of survivors still suffer some degree of paralysis; 35 percent have symptoms of depression; 30 percent need help walking; and 26 percent need help performing daily functions.

Rehabilitation programs can help recover some lost abilities. You can regain to some extent your control over certain muscles, and in some cases learn to speak in an intelligible manner, or move body parts that were paralyzed. But recovery after a major stroke is never complete. Dead neurons do not regenerate. So rehabilitation is not aimed at repairing the brain—which might be possible in the future, but today remains only a hope—and thus rehabilitation is aimed at making the best use of the patient's still-functioning neurons.

CHAPTER TWENTY-THREE

When to See a Cardiologist Even Though It's Not an Emergency

In September 2000, a young woman of twenty-eight collapsed minutes after getting off a plane at Heathrow, having traveled halfway around the world on a twenty-one-hour flight from Melbourne. The attempts to reanimate her were in vain. An autopsy later revealed that she had not had a heart attack but a pulmonary embolism: a large blood clot had broken off from a vein in her leg and blocked the artery that carries blood from the heart to the lungs.

A few days later it became apparent that it is not uncommon for dangerous clots to form in the veins of passengers' legs on intercontinental flights, though the young woman's case was exceptional because she died so suddenly. There is even a name for the condition that killed her: Economy Class Syndrome (ECS), so-called because it mostly affects people flying economy class, where the space between seats is limited, and people remain seated for many hours without moving their legs, so that the blood can become stagnant and clots can form in the veins.

Today, now that the airlines have acknowledged the problem, most passengers on intercontinental flights know that they should move their legs at least every two or three hours to stimulate their circulation and prevent a clot from forming. The young woman who died at Heathrow was the victim of an extreme form of a common problem: poor circulation in the leg veins, a problem that is regarded as minor but can have major consequences. And Economy Class Syndrome is not unique in this sense: in fact, there are a whole range of symptoms in cardiology that, though not emergencies, should be discussed with a specialist.

Peripheral Arterial Disease

Take the example of the person who suffers from pain in their thighs or calves when walking, a pain so intense that they sometimes have to stop. This person may have what we call Peripheral Arterial Disease (PAD), in which the arteries in the legs are partially occluded by atherosclerosis. PAD has nothing to do with poor circulation in the leg veins, which is at the root of Economy Class Syndrome. It is instead related to coronary artery problems such as heart attacks: it is essentially the same problem, but in the legs, not the heart. In fact, it is so closely linked to the heart that we regard it as equivalent to coronary disease because a person with PAD has roughly the same risk of cardiac death as someone who has already had a heart attack.

PAD itself is not fatal, but it indicates that atherosclerosis is so advanced that a heart attack is not far behind. For this reason, one of the most effective strategies we have today for preventing heart attacks is to identify people who suffer from PAD. This is not always easy because there are people who experience pain when walking and do not have PAD, and others who have PAD and walk without pain. Where there is pain in the legs while walking, the problem is to establish whether it is due to PAD or to some other cause, such as arthritis of the hip or compression of nerve fibers in the spine, which can have repercussions below the waist. Though these are different problems, the symptoms are similar, and in some cases the sufferer may have to see several specialists before arriving at a correct diagnosis.

The most effective technique to date for diagnosing PAD is what is called the ankle-brachial index. This simple test consists of simultaneously gauging the blood pressure in the arm and the ankle: if the arterial tension in the ankle is more than 10 percent lower than the pressure in the arm, there is impaired blood flow in the leg. The greater the difference in pressure between ankle and arm, the greater the impairment. This test has the advantage of being so simple that any doctor or nurse can do it at any time; what is more, it is so inexpensive that any health system can afford it, and, above all, it is so effective that it identifies the 70 percent of people with PAD who do not have pain when walking. For all of these reasons, I believe that in the not too distant future this test will be routinely applied to everyone over the age of fifty.

Once PAD has been diagnosed, treatment has two objectives. The first is to halt the advance of atherosclerosis and reduce the risk of a heart attack or other cardiovascular accident by acting on cholesterol, blood pressure, and blood clotting. The second objective is to correct the specific problem in the legs, and for this we advise the patient to try to walk, even if it is painful because walking stimulates the circulation in the legs, and in extreme cases we may implant a stent or bypass sections of damaged artery.

Where these treatments are not applied, or where they prove to be insufficient, and an artery becomes totally occluded, the area of the patient's leg or foot that has stopped receiving blood loses its pulse and is pale, cold, and painful. In these cases, PAD becomes an emergency: an emergency not as urgent as a heart attack because it is not fatal, and we have a few more hours to clear the blockage, but it is essential to act quickly so as to prevent gangrene and the resulting need to amputate the leg.

Diabetes and Metabolic Syndrome

In addition to PAD, two other diseases are regarded as equivalent to a heart condition. The most important in terms of the number of people it affects is diabetes. It is estimated that over 5 percent of the U.S. population, more than 15 million people, suffer from Type 2 diabetes, the most common form, though around half of them do not yet know they are diabetic. In this case, ignorance is a risk: cardiac mortality rates in people with diabetes are similar to those of people who have been diagnosed with heart disease. And if the risk is so high, it is because diabetes is not treated with the seriousness it deserves—all too often it is dismissed as being of secondary importance: the treatments applied are ineffectual, and excessively high levels of glucose in the blood are tolerated—when in fact it is a health problem of the first magnitude.

I am not saying that diabetes ought to be treated by cardiologists. The specialist best equipped to deal with diabetes is the endocrinologist, and it can also, in theory, be treated by the family physician. But it is a complex disease, more complex than hypertension, and there are too many cases in which the measures prescribed by the family doctor are not sufficient to deal with it. When this occurs, it is preferable to refer the patient to a specialist than risk them having a cardiovascular accident that could have been prevented.

Along with diabetes, we have recently begun to attach greater importance to what we call metabolic syndrome, which is often a prelude to Type 2 diabetes. Metabolic syndrome takes in a series of disorders: each of them on its own constitutes an increased cardiovascular risk, and together they make a formidable cocktail. These include abdominal obesity (more than 120 centimeters or 40 inches around the waist in men and more than 80 centimeters or 31 inches in women); excess triglycerides (over 150 milligrams per deciliter of blood); excess blood glucose (over 100 mg/dl on an empty stomach); low HDL cholesterol (less than 40 mg/dl in a man and less than 50 in a woman); and high blood pressure (more than 120 maximum or 80 minimum [Fig. 7]).

Anyone with three or more of these five disorders has metabolic syndrome, as defined by the U.S. National Cholesterol

Education Program. And anyone with metabolic syndrome has a 10 percent risk of cardiovascular mortality within ten years— more than double the risk for the population as a whole.

Aortic Aneurysm

The third equivalent of coronary disease, after PAD and diabetes, is an aortic aneurysm. The aorta is the major artery that carries blood from the heart to the rest of the body, and an aneurysm is a widening of the artery, which bulges like a balloon at a point where the wall of the artery is weakest. A lot of aortic aneurysms are located in the abdomen, through which the blood flows on its way to the legs, but they can also occur in the chest, at the point of exit from the heart. In most cases they are the result of atherosclerosis, and are particularly associated with hypertension and smoking: the more advanced the atherosclerosis, the more likely it is that the aortic artery will deteriorate, with part of it being weak enough for an aneurysm to form.

When an abdominal aneurysm measures less than 4 centimeters in diameter, we recommend periodic checkups to see if it is getting bigger. Where the aneurysm is more than 4 centimeters in diameter, we advise surgery, given the high risk that the artery will burst, resulting in sudden death: less than 20 percent of cases survive more than five years with an abdominal aneurysm of more than 5 centimeters. The operation, which is high risk, consists in reinforcing the aorta by implanting a length of artificial artery at the site of the aneurysm.

One of the major problems with aortic aneurysms is that over 70 percent of those affected do not experience any kind of pain, and of those who do, it is not the same for all. The pain can be mild or severe, constant or intermittent, and only rarely bad enough for the sufferer to decide to see a doctor. As a result, the vast majority of cases are detected only by chance, when the abdomen is examined with an imaging technique in order to diagnose some other ailment.

A good all-around physician who knows how to explore a patient's abdomen with their hands can detect an aortic aneurysm by touch, and given that this is a very common problem, affecting perhaps 2 percent of the population, it is not a bad idea to feel the abdomen of a patient with hypertension or atherosclerosis to check for a potential aneurysm. However, the fact is that nowadays most aneurysms are not found by touch but with imaging techniques, so that in a significant proportion of cases they remain undiagnosed and are not discovered until the artery bursts, causing a massive hemorrhage.

Chronic Angina Pectoris

One disease that does directly affect the heart is chronic angina. This is perceived as a crushing pain in the center of the chest and can extend, as with heart attack, to the entire chest, the arms (usually the left arm), the neck, the jaw, the back, and the pit of the stomach. But unlike the acute pain of a heart attack, angina is a recurrent pain (Fig. 10); it appears in situations of physical exertion or emotional stress and eases with rest and calm. In most cases, the pain is caused by the coronary arteries being narrowed by atherosclerosis but not totally occluded, as they are in a heart attack. Angina pectoris can be likened to driving on a very narrow road: the traffic does not flow smoothly, and the risk of an accident is heightened.

The problem is particularly apparent at moments of effort or stress, when the heart has to pump blood with greater intensity than in a state of repose, which is like driving even faster on that very narrow road. What happens then is that the heart does not receive enough oxygen via the coronary arteries for it to beat with the required intensity, so it has to resort to an alternative form of energy production that does not need oxygen. Result: the heart does its job because it is capable of burning glucose without oxygen, but in so doing it produces lactic acid, which is a painful residue. The pain caused by the lactic acid—the same substance that causes pain during a heart attack or when we make too great a physical effort—is the signal that the heart is working beyond its capacity.

Though angina is a disease of the coronary arteries, it is rarely an emergency. In most cases, it remains stable for years, making certain activities uncomfortable or painful but not putting the patient's life in danger. Only in those cases where the angina becomes unstable, with intense intermittent pain that lasts a few minutes and is not the result of any special overstrain, is it advisable to go to the emergency room because it may be the prelude to a heart attack.

With angina, the paradox is that more or less intense pain does not mean that the disease is more or less advanced. There are people who experience great pain and are not in any imminent danger, and vice versa: there are high-risk patients who have very little pain. In fact, 25 percent of patients who have the conditions for angina because their coronary arteries are dangerously narrowed, do not feel any discomfort. To detect this 25 percent, anyone who may have a significant risk of insufficient blood flow in the heart should be given a stress test.

Treatment usually starts with dilating drugs to increase the diameter of the coronary arteries and improve the blood flow, or with beta-blockers, which allow the heart to function with less oxygen. When medication is not sufficient—this mostly applies to young patients whom the pain is preventing from doing their preferred form of physical activity—the usual procedure is to introduce a stent or do a bypass to restore proper circulation in the heart.

Damaged Valves

Other forms of cardiac disease, but not coronary disease, affect the heart valves (Fig. 11). The function of the heart valves is to keep the blood moving forward in its passage through the four cavities of the heart—the two atria above and the two ventricles below—and prevent it from coming to a standstill or flowing backward. This is not a simple journey: oxygen-poor blood arrives in the right atrium of the heart by way of two major veins, passes from there to the right ventricle, is sent to the lungs to be oxygenated, returns to the heart via the left atrium, passes down into the left ventricle and finally emerges, rich in oxygen, from the aortic valve (Fig. 11).

In order for this process to run smoothly, the heart has four valves, which act like traffic lights. They open up to let the blood flow through and then close, briefly retaining the blood inside the heart. But one or another of these four valves—aortic, mitral, pulmonary, and tricuspid—can malfunction and cause traffic problems in the heart. If a valve is too tight—what we call a stenosis—it hampers forward blood flow, like having a green light and finding that one of the lanes is blocked off. If, on the other hand, a valve is too open, and suffers from what is known as valvular insufficiency, it lets the blood flow backward, and the effect is like facing a red light and having the traffic in front trying to reverse: a guaranteed jam.

What patients are most aware of in such cases is shortness of breath when they make any kind of physical effort, however small because the blood in the lungs is stagnant and they feel they have to overcome a great deal of resistance when they breathe in. Though valvular disease rarely becomes critical, without proper treatment it can degenerate into cardiac failure and become fatal, either because the sufferer has so much difficulty breathing that they suffocate or because the heart, unable to meet the demands made by the body, goes into an irreversible arrhythmia.

Treatment usually starts with diuretic drugs, which reduce the amount of blood that the heart has to handle—and which may be stagnating in the lungs: the heart needs to make less effort, and the feeling of suffocation is eased. In some cases—especially with mitral stenosis—a valve that is too tight can be opened up by inserting a catheter in the thigh and feeding it back through the arteries to the heart. But in the majority of serious cases, surgery is necessary, either to repair the damaged valve or to replace it with a biological or mechanical valve. The biological valves, usually from a pig's or sheep's heart, have the advantage of not requiring subsequent treatment with anticoagulants but the disadvantage of needing to be replaced every few years.

Heart Failure

Heart failure occurs when the heart's ability to pump blood is no longer sufficient for the body's needs. The patient feels shortness of breath, sometimes even when lying down, and gets tired at the least effort. Other symptoms include swelling of the feet and legs, discomfort in the upper abdomen caused by the accumulation of blood in the liver, and sometimes a loss of appetite and nausea. Heart failure can be a result of valvular disease, a heart attack (where a significant amount of heart tissue has been destroyed), or a cardiomyopathy (a disease of the heart muscle). In all three cases, the heart is unequal to its task and is forced to overexert itself to pump blood with its limited resources.

Though heart failure is a serious illness which in some cases requires a heart transplant, we have drugs and informed advice that serve to keep the problem under control in a high percentage of patients. The most useful drugs are the diuretics, which reduce the amount of blood the heart has to deal with and control blood pressure because high blood pressure makes the heart contract more forcefully. The key pieces of advice include not drinking too much (because alcohol interferes with the heart's ability to contract), keeping an eye on salt consumption (to reduce the volume of blood and hypertension), and going to the doctor if you have a constant or progressive feeling of suffocation.

figure 11

EXTERIOR AND INTERIOR VIEW OF THE HEART

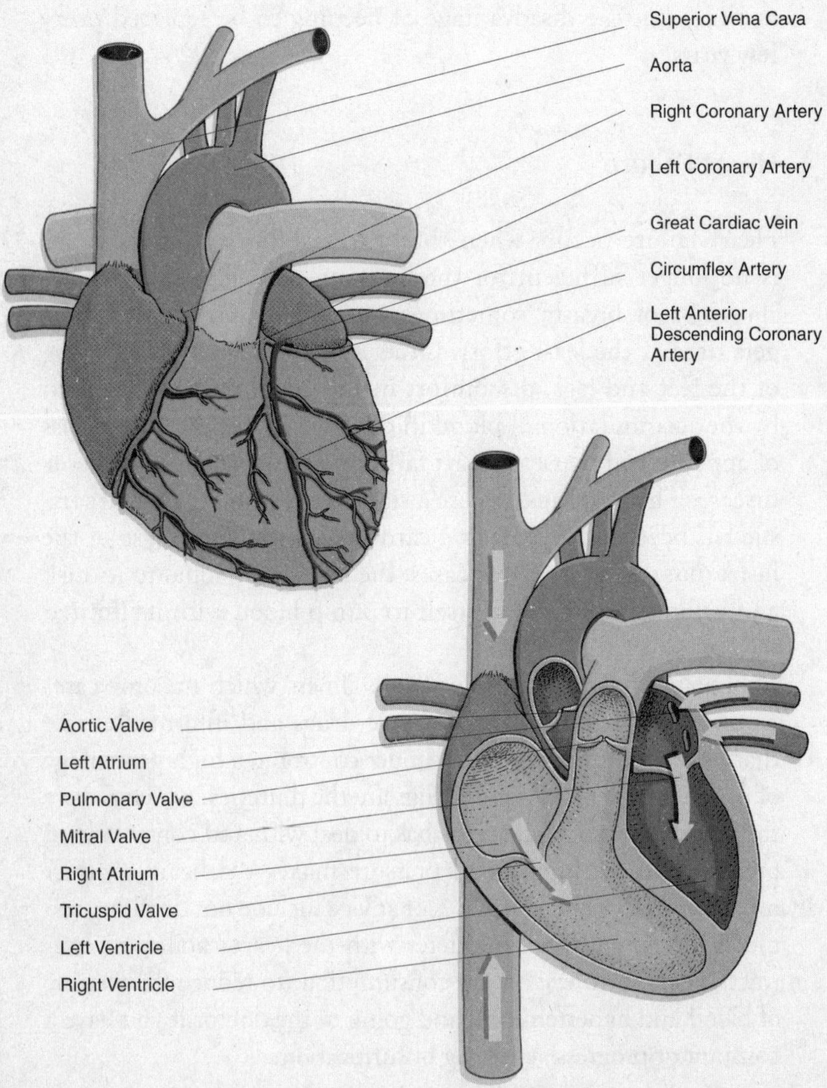

Superior Vena Cava

Aorta

Right Coronary Artery

Left Coronary Artery

Great Cardiac Vein

Circumflex Artery

Left Anterior Descending Coronary Artery

Aortic Valve

Left Atrium

Pulmonary Valve

Mitral Valve

Right Atrium

Tricuspid Valve

Left Ventricle

Right Ventricle

Arrhythmias

Heart failure, and indeed any disease that affects the heart, can lead to an arrhythmia. An arrhythmia is an alteration in the rhythm of the heart's contractions, and this can take various forms. Often it is felt as palpitations in the chest—most of which are temporary and harmless. For example, the pulse can be abnormally fast (tachycardia, though most tachycardias are not arrhythmias) or abnormally slow (bradycardia), or irregular and rapid (atrial fibrillation); the pulse can stop in cardiac arrest (ventricular fibrillation) or from a fault in the heart's electrical signal (heart block). Most cases of arrhythmia are benign, and almost all respond to treatment if diagnosed in time.

So, when a patient comes to see us with an arrhythmia, the first thing we do is find out what kind of arrhythmia they have, in order to decide on the appropriate treatment. Above all, we need to know which part of the heart it originates in, and whether it has appeared spontaneously or is a consequence of some other disease. Let us look at three examples.

The most common arrhythmia is atrial fibrillation, which affects one in every twenty people aged over seventy and is usually benign. It originates in the atria—the upper chambers of the heart—and patients note that their heartbeats are irregular and rapid. The treatment is based on drugs to slow down and stabilize the heart's rhythm and is often supplemented with anticoagulants.

Much less frequent but more serious is ventricular tachycardia, which originates in the ventricles (the lower chambers of the heart) and can degenerate into ventricular fibrillation and sudden death. We have drugs to treat the problem and in high-risk patients we implant an electric defibrillator under the skin to restore the electrical signal that makes the heart beat in the event of cardiac arrest.

With bradycardia we are dealing with the opposite situation. The heart beats so slowly that the sufferer may pass out because not enough blood is getting to the brain. The origin of the problem is usually in the heart's natural pacemaker, the two groups of cells that regulate the beating of the heart. The usual treatment in such cases is to introduce an artificial pacemaker to take control of the situation.

Varicosis: Thrombi in the Veins and Pulmonary Embolism

There is a further significant valvular disease, one which affects not the heart but the valves in the legs: varicose veins. In the legs, the blood circulates through the arteries in the downward direction, and once its oxygen has been consumed, the veins carry it back up to the heart and lungs for recycling. However, this poses a complicated engineering problem: how to overcome the force of gravity so that the blood that is trying to climb back up to the heart is not pushed back down to the feet by the weight of all the blood above it.

The solution nature came up with is to have valves in the veins so that the blood moves in only one direction and cannot flow backward. However, many of us find that these valves tend to deteriorate with age and the blood becomes stagnant in thickened veins that protrude and are sometimes painful. And though many people think of their varicose veins as primarily an aesthetic problem, they carry a risk of two more serious problems that affect circulation in the legs: thrombophlebitis and deep vein thrombosis.

Thrombophlebitis is when a blood clot forms on the wall of a vein. When the vein is superficial—just beneath the skin—the area is red and inflamed, and painful to the touch. Most of these superficial cases are unimportant, and there is no need to see a doctor unless the thrombophlebitis persists for more than two or three days or the symptoms are severe or get worse.

More serious, and also more difficult to detect, is deep vein thrombosis. Though the problem is similar to thrombophlebitis—the formation of a blood clot in a vein—it always originates in blood vessels that are not accessible to the touch and carries a risk of pulmonary embolism. This was what killed the young woman at Heathrow Airport just after a twenty-one-hour flight. Especially vulnerable to deep vein thrombosis and pulmonary embolism are people who are confined to bed for a long time, for example, after a hip operation: in such cases specific preventive treatment with compression stockings and anticoagulants is advisable.

There have also been cases in which, unlike the Heathrow incident, the thrombosis complications did not appear immediately after a long journey but two or three days later. So if someone has a feeling of suffocation after a long plane journey, it is worth bearing in mind that it could be a pulmonary embolism caused by the breaking off of a blood clot that formed in their leg during the flight. More than half the cases of deep vein thrombosis occur without any telltale symptoms. In others, there may be a feeling of discomfort in the legs, especially when walking, but very few people connect the sensation with thrombosis.

As there are no symptoms to enable effective early diagnosis, prevention is based on stimulating the circulation in the legs so as to reduce the risk of clots forming: we should avoid standing or sitting still for too long without moving our legs. For example, on a long flight, it is a good idea to get out of your seat and walk up and down for a while every couple of hours. And it is often recommended to people who have varicose veins, or who spend several hours a day standing or sitting without moving, to wear knee-length elastic stockings to help the valves in their leg veins do their job.

CHAPTER TWENTY-FOUR

Longevity

HOW LONG CAN WE GET TO LIVE?

I do not think there is any piece of engineering in the world more perfect than the heart. I have spent more than thirty-five years studying it, and I still do not understand how it can beat 100,000 times a day, in some cases for more than one hundred years, without stopping for a single second, without wearing out, and without deforming as any other muscle would. A Boeing 747 may seem like a miracle of engineering, but every few weeks it goes into the hangar for maintenance. The Hubble Space Telescope has revealed hitherto unsuspected mysteries of the universe, but it has had to be repaired five times since it was put into orbit in 1990.

As a triumph of engineering, a heart is way above an airplane, a space telescope, or the most sophisticated rocket. There is no law, no satisfactory physical or chemical explanation, to help us understand how a heart can pump 17,000 pints of blood a day, from before birth until death. Of all the wonders of the heart, the most intriguing is that it does not wear out. It can break down if we abuse it with an excess of fats or drugs or if it suffers some accidental infection. But if we respect it, it can maintain its ability to keep on steadily beating for eighty, ninety, even one hundred years.

There are species of turtle—though these are animals whose biology is very different from ours, of course—in which the heart goes on beating for more than two hundred years. And the inevitable question, when we stop to think about the wonder of the human heart, is how many years it could carry on beating. How long can we get to live?

Toward a Life Expectancy of More Than One Hundred Years

The immediate answer to that question is that no one knows. However, if we look at the evolution of life expectancy in the developed countries, we find that for the last fifteen decades it has consistently kept on increasing at a rate of more than two years per decade. Every claim that we had reached the definitive upper limit beyond which we cannot go has been refuted by the facts: one after another, every supposed limit has been exceeded. It is very probable that there is a biological limit to human longevity, but if there is, it is not on the horizon yet.

If we were nearing the limit, the increase in life expectancy ought to be slowing down. And it is not; in the last thirty years, the average lifetime has lengthened by more than six years—the same rate as in the previous one hundred years.

So I do not know how long we may be able to live, but I do not think it unreasonable to assume that as medicine continues to progress in the decades to come, life expectancy may continue to rise by between two and three years per decade, may reach one hundred years in the middle of this century, the most long-lived people may carry on to the age of one hundred twenty-five, and many children born in the last decade of the twentieth century may live to welcome in the twenty-second century.

In the longer term, it is possible that human life could be extended even further. The longevity of a species is built into its genetic code. This is what determines that a butterfly will live a single spring, a dog fifteen years, an elephant sixty, or a turtle more than two hundred: by manipulating a few genes, nature has adapted the life cycle of each species to its reproductive cycle, so that every living being has the best chance of leaving offspring. That is how death works because that is how life works. It all stems from a sophisticated program of reproduction.

And the kind of genetic manipulation that nature engages in is being tested in laboratories, where biologists investigating longevity prolong the life of worms and flies by experimenting with a few genes. It is possible that someday this research will help prolong human life. I do not know. But if it does, it will certainly not be easy, and it will certainly not be soon. For now, what seems to be an achievable goal in the medium term is that living to one hundred will cease to be exceptional and become fairly normal, at least in the developed countries. The big question, of course, is how to reach that goal and how to maintain the quality of life (i.e., problems with dementia, depression, Parkinson's disease, etc.).

Some studies suggest that the key may lie in consuming fewer calories. In experiments with flies, worms, and even mice—which, as mammals, have a biology similar to ours—a nutritious, balanced diet that is low in calories has proved to prolong life. However, it is questionable whether the results of these experiments can be applied to human beings, where a low body mass index does not prolong life but increases the risk of premature death. The fact is that the highest survival rates are found in the ideal weight range, among people with a body mass index of between 18.5 and 25. Until further research into longevity genes or reducing our calorie intake manages to establish why we age, the best we can do for now to slow the decline of aging is to keep ourselves active, both physically and mentally.

A whole host of studies show that people who continue to engage in mentally stimulating activities as they grow older— activities such as reading, playing chess, and playing music— tend to stay lucid until a much greater age than those who lapse into monotony. It seems as if the brain behaves similarly to a muscle: if you exercise it, it stays in shape; if you stop exercising it, it atrophies.

There is also a mass of research to show that physically active people tend to stay agile, independent, and in good health for longer than sedentary people: again, inactivity accelerates atrophy. We have yet to discover what happens in our cells when we make an effort, whether physical or mental, in order to understand why it is that effort should act as an antidote to aging. But we know that aging is related to the process by which cells self-destruct, which is known as apoptosis, or programmed cell death.

My hypothesis, on the basis of the data we have, is that cells do not always self-destruct because too much is demanded of them and they are overwhelmed, but in many cases because too little is demanded of them. Here again, the example of the muscle comes to mind: when muscle cells are active, they remain vigorous; when they lapse into inactivity, they deteriorate. It is as if the cells were saying: "Okay, we're not needed here—let's take ourselves out of circulation."

Medicine Will Transform Society

Enabling the majority of the population to live for one hundred years would be a remarkable breakthrough, but the implications of that development for society, and for the way we practice medicine, may entail major conflicts. The most obvious of these is the increase in the number of people over sixty-five as a proportion of the population as a whole. Those over sixty-five already constitute the fastest-growing section of the population in the developed countries. And this poses a major economic problem: How does a society in which the non-active population is steadily increasing thanks to medical progress sustain itself? How do we pay rising health-care costs for the elderly if the proportion of people working to cover these costs is dwindling?

Fortunately, the progress of medical science not only raises the problem but also offers a solution. When the retirement age was set at sixty-five, most people of that age were regarded as old, and it was not uncommon for people to die before they reached seventy. Today, if someone dies in their sixties, we think of them as dying young. Most people now arrive at retirement age in full possession of their physical and mental faculties, perfectly able to carry on contributing to society.

If life expectancy is to continue to rise without the system collapsing, the only solution is to give people the opportunity to contribute to society beyond the age of sixty-five. One option would be to raise the retirement age. An alternative, or a complementary option, would be for retired people to be recruited into the social welfare services or provide other kinds of service to the community. This is already being done, for example, by older people who look after their grandchildren while the parents are at work. Or by those retired people who take on the running of their local residence association.

But these initiatives involving a minority of people from a minority of families will not be sufficient to sustain the system. If life expectancy continues to rise in the years ahead—and I do not know anyone who is opposed to the idea—we will have to rethink the role of those over sixty-five in society. Of course, it will not be easy: a lot of people, both employers and employees, are happy with the retirement age as it is today. But unless we find some formula to allow people to continue to contribute to the community for as long as they are able—and I hope that we do—we are going to find ourselves in a very difficult situation. There will be treatments to save sick people, but we will not be able to afford them.

Longevity or Quality of Life?

If we do not resolve this question of the role of the elderly in society, we are heading for a future in which the progress of medicine will be limited because what may be possible at the theoretical level may not be economically viable. And what will limit the increase in life expectancy will not be science but economics.

To some extent this is already starting to happen. In Britain, the public health service no longer covers certain treatments that save lives but are considered too expensive. We have the knowledge to develop new therapies to cure old diseases, but we are not investing in them because they are unlikely to be profitable. Clinical trials of new diagnostic techniques and new drugs not only look at whether they are effective in curing disease or prolonging life. They also analyze their cost, and I think that soon they will also take into account whether they effectively improve the patient's quality of life.

What this all goes to show is that medicine is entering a new phase in its history. The goal of preventing disease and premature death is still a priority, and much of the advice given in this book is directed to that goal. But having reduced premature mortality, as we are doing for large sections of the population, the emphasis shifts from survival and longevity—what we might call the quantity of life—to the quality of life.

Imagine for a moment that we succeed in our efforts to prevent and treat cardiovascular disease. That cancer research results in new treatments capable of curing the disease as completely as antibiotics today cure infections that were fatal less than a century ago. That we find effective treatments for Alzheimer's, as we may do in a decade or so. What will the goal of medicine be then?

I believe the day will come when physicians will work to ensure that the human body completes its life cycle, suffering the minimum possible burden of disease and enjoying the highest possible quality of life, and that death comes at the end, not from disease but from the aging of the organism itself. And I believe this will lead us to rethink other priorities, such as the importance we attach to longevity.

Until now, longevity was the priority: starting from the fact that we are all born with the instinct of not wanting to die, since its inception medicine has tried to cure disease, which has allowed us to live longer, and greater longevity has been a reflection of the success of medicine. But the most important thing is not to live longer: what really matters is to live well.

With present-day technology we can keep people alive, sometimes for a long time, even though they may have a very poor quality of life and no prospect of recovery. Personally, I do not believe this is a rational use of technology. I believe that there must be a point where we learn to say "enough." I do not know where that point ought to be, but we can no longer let ourselves be guided solely by the principle of maximum survival.

Future Solidarity

What medicine will achieve if it succeeds in ensuring a good quality of life for the elderly is not only that they feel well and enjoy their longevity, which is a noble goal, but also that they can continue to contribute to the community, which is even nobler. The idea has never been that a few people should take advantage of what society has to offer them—in this case, advances in medicine—without offering anything in return. We humans are a social species, and this is in origin the fundamental rule of the game: others help us and we help others. The problem is that the evolution of capitalism has not always led us in this direction, but frequently in the opposite direction, toward a ferocious individualism. And there is a real danger that medical advances in decades to come, possibly resulting in more expensive diagnostic techniques and treatments than those we have today, will not lead to greater solidarity but to greater inequalities, in which some people—or some countries—are able to afford technologies that are unattainable for others.

To assume that inequalities are an inevitable side effect of technological progress seems to me to be an exercise in cynicism. Personally, I am convinced that an increase in inequality is a risk we cannot afford. A future of peace and prosperity will depend on reducing inequalities, both within countries and among countries. That is why we in the West cannot be satisfied with medicine's ability to prevent and cure the diseases that have become the principal causes of death among us: we must actively involve ourselves in eradicating poverty and infectious diseases in the poorer countries.

If we are not willing to do this from altruism, perhaps we will be persuaded to do it from selfishness because otherwise the tensions between rich and poor will only intensify, and in a globalized world in which millions of people have access to technologies of destruction, the results are impossible to predict.

It is not only the progress of medicine that leads inevitably to profound social changes, changes affecting the role that older people play in the community and, possibly, the way we manage our wealth and show our solidarity. Along with medical advances, changes in other fields such as IT, electronics, transport, or our relationship with the environment leave us no alternative but to evolve toward a new model of society—a society that will only be viable and peaceful if it transcends its present individualism and is based on cooperation.

This may sound like a utopia, but it is not an impossible task: the tendency to cooperate, to help one another, is part of the program with which we humans are born. The great unknown is whether the transition to this new society will be traumatic or if, instead, we will succeed in putting aside our selfishness and make a smooth transition.

Emergency Dictionary

Angina. A chest pain, usually during exercise, related to the obstruction of coronary arteries that deprives the heart muscle of blood when it is most needed (i.e., exercise).

Angioplasty. A technique for opening occluded arteries that consists in introducing a small deflated balloon inside the artery with a catheter and inflating it at the site of the occlusion, so that the artery is opened up by the outward pressure of the balloon. To prevent the artery re-occluding, a small mesh cylinder called a stent is implanted inside it (Fig. 10).

Aorta. This is the large artery that carries blood from the heart at the start of its circulation around the body.

Arrhythmia. An alteration of the regular contractions of the heart. The two most common types of arrhythmia are tachycardia (abnormally rapid pulse, though not all tachycardias are arrhythmias) and bradycardia (abnormally slow pulse).

Arteries and veins. These are the two types of vessels through which the blood circulates around the body. The arteries carry oxygenated blood on its outward journey from the heart to the various organs of the body. The veins carry blood back to the heart once the oxygen has been used up.

Atherosclerosis. A disease in which the walls of the arteries thicken and lose their elasticity. Atherosclerosis is due to the buildup of fat and other deposits on the walls of the arteries, narrowing the interior of the blood vessel.

Bypass. A surgical intervention to restore the circulation in a blocked artery. It involves grafting a section of blood vessel onto the artery to form a bridge so that the blood can flow past the obstruction (Fig. 10).

Carotid artery. These are the two large arteries inside the neck that carry blood to the head (See illustration on page 247).

Catheter. A sterile flexible tube inserted into the body as part of a diagnosis or treatment. Vascular catheters, which are usually introduced by way of a blood vessel in the leg, arm, or neck, provide access to the heart (Fig. 10).

Coronary arteries. These are the small arteries that take blood to the heart muscle (Fig. 6).

Coronary heart disease. Atherosclerosis in the arteries of the heart.

Coronary heart disease equivalent. A condition in which the risk of heart disease in the future is as high as it is for people suffering from coronary disease.

Defibrillator. A device that applies an electric shock to the heart to restore its ability to beat in the event of cardiac arrest.

Electrocardiogram. Graphic monitoring of the electrical activity of the heart. It causes no discomfort and is very useful for diagnosing heart disease.

Embolism. Occlusion of an artery by something—almost always a clot, but it can also be a particle of calcium or fat or an air bubble—carried in the bloodstream.

Endothelium. The fine layer of cells that covers the inner walls of blood vessels and other body cavities.

Glycemia. The level of glucose (or sugar) in the blood.

HDL cholesterol. Good cholesterol: the more you have, the better. This is not cholesterol in its pure state but a protein that carries cholesterol in the blood. HDL has a high proportion of protein to cholesterol. Because the protein weighs more than the cholesterol, it has a high density. The initials HDL stand for high-density lipoprotein.

Heart attack. See myocardial infraction.

Insulin. The hormone that regulates glucose levels in blood to prevent them from rising above or falling below the acceptable level.

LDL cholesterol. Bad cholesterol: the less you have, the better. In reality, this is a protein that contains a large amount of cholesterol. The initials LDL stand for low-density lipoprotein.

Metabolic syndrome. A group of symptoms that are often the prelude to Type 2 diabetes: abdominal obesity, excess triglycerides, excess blood glucose, HDL cholesterol deficiency, and high blood pressure. A person who has any three of these five symptoms is considered to have metabolic syndrome.

Myocardial infarction. The death of part of the heart muscle due to its being deprived of blood by the occlusion of a coronary artery (Fig. 6).

Myocardium. The heart muscle; the technical name comes from the Greek roots *mus*, meaning muscle, and *kardia*, meaning heart.

Pacemaker. A healthy heart has a natural pacemaker formed by groups of cells that regulate its beating. If this fails, an artificial pacemaker may be implanted to tell the heart when to beat.

Statins. Drugs prescribed to reduce the level of LDL cholesterol. They also have an anti-inflammatory action.

Stent. A small mesh cylinder implanted in a clogged artery to keep it open. They are usually from 1 to 3 centimeters long and between 3 and 4 millimeters in diameter (Fig. 10).

Stroke. Cerebral vascular accident in which there is a massive destruction of neurons. It may be caused by obstruction of a blood vessel in the brain or by a hemorrhage.

Thrombosis. The formation of a clot inside a blood vessel (Fig. 6).

Triglycerides. A type of fat the human body uses to store energy and as a fuel for the muscles that can also increase cardiovascular risk.

Type 1 diabetes. A disease in which the body is unable to regulate the level of glucose in the blood because the cells in the pancreas that produce insulin have been destroyed. It usually first appears in childhood or adolescence. Type 1 is the most serious, but less common, form of diabetes.

Type 2 diabetes. A disease in which the body cannot regulate the level of glucose in the blood adequately because its insulin is no longer working properly. Generally associated with obesity, it usually first appears in adulthood.

VLDL cholesterol. Usually included in the cholesterol group, VLDL is a protein that contains a small portion of the triglycerides in the blood, rather than a type of cholesterol. Like LDL, an excess of triglycerides and VLDL is harmful. VLDL stands for very low-density lipoprotein.

Index

fructose, 135, 136
fruit
  antioxidants in, 98, 99–100, 102
  choosing by color, 100–101
  decline in consumption, 103–104, 139
  dried, 107, 117
  fiber and, 101–102
  in food pyramid, 107
  ideal amount per day, 103, 138
  simple carbohydrates and, 135, 136, 139
fruit juices, 134, 139

gallstones, 47
garlic, antioxidants in, 98, 103
gastoenteritis, 91
gastric cancers, 115, 128, 154
gender
  alcohol metabolism and use, 148–152
  cardiovascular disease and, 8, 37, 222–223
  exercise and, 8–9, 174
  Framingham risk factor scale, 39–40
  impact of atherosclerosis on sexual performance, 213–215
  reaction to heart attack symptoms, 222–223
  smoking and, 155
genetic factors
  in atherosclerosis, 241
  in hypercholesterolemia, 69–70
  as risk factor for cardiovascular disease, 24
  in weight problems, 43, 55–56
glucose, 135. *See also* blood glucose
glucosinolate, 101
glycemia test, 27, 34
gout, 123–124

grafts, in bypass surgery, 232
Greece
  health problems, 4
  Mediterranean diet, 4
green beans, 104
grilling food, 119
gym, in school curriculum, 18

hake, 126, 127
half portions, at restaurants, 57
hallucinogens, 21, 217
hamburger, 124
Harvard University, 170
hazelnuts, 99, 112, 129
HDL cholesterol (High-Density Lipoprotein/good cholesterol), 32–33, 46, 65
  alcohol in raising, 144–145
  antioxidant effects, 68
  ideal levels, 68–69
  monounsaturated fats in raising, 111
  polyunsaturated fats in reducing, 112
  role in body, 68
  strategies for raising, 15, 69–70, 71–72, 73, 111, 144–145, 166, 171, 172, 181–182
headache
  chronic stress and, 195
  hypertension and, 82
  as stroke symptom, 251
heart
  alcohol impact on, 149
  anatomy of, 266
  hypertension and, 78
heart attack, 105, 221–234
  acute stress and, 189–192
  alcohol in preventing, 149–150
  anatomy of, 67, 89, 223
  childhood habits and, 12–13